The Athletic Trainer's Pocket Guide to
Clinical Teaching

Thomas G. Weidner, PhD, ATC, FNATA
Director, Athletic Training Education Program
Director, Athletic Training Research & Education Laboratory
Professor of Athletic Training, School of Physical Education,
Sport and Exercise Science
Ball State University
Muncie, Indiana

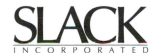

SLACK
INCORPORATED

Published by: SLACK Incorporated
                  6900 Grove Road
                  Thorofare, NJ 08086 USA
                  Telephone: 856-848-1000
                  Fax: 856-848-6091
                  www.slackbooks.com

Contact SLACK Incorporated for more information about other books in this field or about the availability of our books from distributors outside the United States.

Library of Congress Cataloging-in-Publication Data

Weidner, Thomas G.
  The athletic trainer's pocket guide to clinical teaching / Thomas G. Weidner.
      p. ; cm.
  Includes bibliographical references and index.
  ISBN 978-1-55642-869-2 (softcover : alk. paper) 1. Athletic trainers--Handbooks, manuals, etc. 2. Sports medicine--Study and teaching--Handbooks, manuals, etc. I. Title.
  [DNLM: 1. Sports Medicine--education--Handbooks. 2. Allied Health Personnel--education--Handbooks. 3. Clinical Competence--Handbooks. 4. Models, Educational--Handbooks. 5. Teaching--methods--Handbooks. QT 29 W418a 2009]
  RC1210.W45 2009
  617.1'027--dc22
                              2009014860

DEDICATION

This handbook is dedicated to those athletic trainers who serve as Approved Clinical Instructors, and to the young professionals you are developing, who will become the future of the athletic training profession.

CONTENTS

SECTION III: CLOSING THE LOOP

APPENDICES

ACKNOWLEDGMENTS

I would like to thank my wife, Lauren Bishop-Weidner, for her support and guidance throughout my career. Also, many thanks to my athletic training colleagues at Ball State University who extend much kindness and encouragement to me.

About the Author

Thomas G. Weidner, PhD, ATC, FNATA completed his undergraduate and graduate studies in Health Education at Southern Illinois University—Carbondale. After serving as the men's assistant athletic trainer at SIU—C, Weidner accepted a position as Director of the Athletic Training Education Program at California State University—Northridge. For the past 18 years at Ball State University, he has served as Coordinator of Clinical Education, Program Director, and Director of the Athletic Training Research and Education Laboratory. Weidner has been professionally involved in NATA and NATA-District 4 service in the areas of professional education and research for many years, including leading and presenting the CIE Seminars for the last 7 years. The recipient of several national and district awards in the NATA, including Distinguished Educator, Weidner continues to conduct, publish, and present research regarding athletic training clinical education.

Contributing Authors

Mary G. Barnum, EdD, ATC, LAT
(Chapter 9)
Director, Athletic Training Education
  Program
Associate Professor, Exercise Science
  and Sport Studies
Springfield College
Springfield, MA

Carrie Graham, MA, ATC, LAT
(Chapter 9)
Clinical Coordinator/Instructor
Entry-Level Athletic Training Education
  Program
Department of Kinesiology
University of Connecticut
Storrs, CT

M. Susan Guyer, DPE, ATC, LAT, CSCS
(Chapter 9)
Clinical Coordinator, Springfield College
Athletic Training Education Program
Assistant Professor, Exercise Science and
  Sport Studies
Springfield College
Springfield, MA

Jolene M. Henning, EdD, ATC, LAT
(Chapters 4, 5, 8, & 10)
Director, Entry-Level Masters Athletic
  Training Education Program
Department of Exercise and Sport
  Science
University of North Carolina Greensboro
Greensboro, NC

Lisa S. Jutte, PhD, ATC, LAT
(Chapter 6)
Assistant Professor of Athletic Training
School of Physical Education, Sport and
  Exercise Science
Ball State University
Muncie, IN

Linda S. Levy, EdD, ATC
(Chapter 9)
Chair, Department of Health and Human
  Performance
Athletic Training Program Director
Plymouth State University
Plymouth, NH

Stacy E. Walker, PhD, ATC, LAT
(Chapter 6)
Assistant Professor of Athletic Training
School of Physical Education, Sport and
  Exercise Science
Ball State University
Muncie, IN

PREFACE

Athletic training clinical education can be described as the portion of professional preparation that involves formal acquisition, practice, and evaluation of clinical proficiencies through classroom, laboratory, and clinical experiences in medical care environments. Clinical education progresses from general technical skills to clinical competence, and students must learn to appreciate the affective aspects of their profession's distinctive working environment as well, developing appropriate social skills and attitudes. Entry-level certified athletic trainers perceive that slightly over half of their entry-level professional development comes from clinical education. Thus, the clinical instructor, identified as the person most critical to the students' learning, plays a vital role in athletic training education.

In a setting dominated by patient care, clinicians are often so busy with patients that they are unable to devote sufficient time and effort to the professional education of students. In the past, clinical educators may have focused efforts on initiating students into the profession socially, teaching through example more than through purposeful instruction, sometimes using students as a labor force for care provision.

In the recent decade, however, clinical education in athletic training has become more structured, progressing from somewhat haphazard learning experiences to deliberate, focused learning experiences. Responsibilities of the student, clinical instructor, and clinical education setting have become more clearly understood and delineated.

Nevertheless, few athletic trainers have received formal instruction regarding clinical supervision and teaching, skills which may or may not come naturally to even the most competent patient care provider. This textbook provides valuable information and resources for Approved Clinical Instructors to effectively and efficiently instruct students during clinical experiences, while maintaining their primary roles as patient care providers.

INTRODUCTION

This book is primarily intended for the athletic training Approved Clinical Instructor (ACI) who teaches and evaluates students' clinical proficiencies and who supervises their clinical experiences. As well, it is ideally suited for athletic training Clinical Instructor Educators (CIEs) who train, develop, and evaluate ACIs. Certainly, it contains beneficial content for any clinical instructor involved in supervising and teaching athletic training students.

The book contains three sections. The first provides chapters with general information about athletic training clinical instruction and supervision, pertinent and relevant learning theories/styles regarding clinical education, and important steps to incorporate and teach evidence-based medicine/practice. One chapter in this section is devoted to ACI training, aimed at those CIEs who are charged with this task. This chapter includes a specially-designed worksheet to assist in capturing essential messages and delivery techniques for this training. The second section contains chapters regarding effective teaching and learning in the clinical setting. This section includes practical, creative, and time-efficient methods and ideas for teaching and supervising athletic training students during their clinical experiences. The third section contains chapters for closing the loop with athletic training students, including evaluation and feedback, and working with difficult students and tough learning situations. Each chapter concludes with reflection questions and suggestions for future improvements, designed to help ACIs understand and refine current teaching practices. Finally, a number of appendices provide working models and resources associated with various roles and responsibilities of ACIs and CIEs.

FOREWORD

Although students learn the science, research, theory, and facts of athletic training in the classroom, they hone their skills and develop professional practice patterns in their clinical experiences. The actual process of watching and engaging in patient care leaves an indelible impression on how students should practice their profession, shaping their attitudes and molding their affective traits. Classroom information builds knowledge, but clinical education experience builds professionals.

Just as people are not automatically good classroom instructors, the mere interaction with students does not mean quality clinical instruction. As with your other professional skills, your development into a quality clinical instructor takes learning, practice, and time.

Dr. Weidner's text, *The Athletic Trainer's Pocket Guide to Clinical Teaching*, provides a practical—and much needed—method for improving the methodology of clinical education and increasing your effectiveness as a clinical instructor. In addition to delivering the "nuts and bolts" of the how, when, and why of clinical education, this text covers topics that are often overlooked or underemphasized in clinical education.

The process of clinical instruction is often lost. Like any form of education, clinical education involves repeated feedback loops, goal setting, and the gradual modeling and synthesis of psychomotor skills, cognitive knowledge, and decision-making skills. Much of this text is devoted to this process and offers you strategies that should be incorporated into your clinical teaching and supervision. An important—and personally meaningful—topic is that of balancing student supervision with autonomy in decision making. When the Education Council first began to revise our clinical education construct, we attempted to emphasize that supervision and autonomy are not dichotomous, a goal we fell far short of. Skill and patience are required to learn to recognize the fine line between allowing the student to err and protecting the patient.

The chapters that discuss the need to incorporate evidence-based practice and the influence of our various practice venues are vital to the advancement of our professional practice. By emphasizing the need for "science" in our professional practice and introducing the nuances of various practice settings, you can help better prepare our students to enter a more diverse range of employment settings.

This text should be a staple for all who are engaged in the clinical education of our students. Our future professional practice will only be as strong as our clinical education.

Chad Starkey, PhD, LAT, FNATA
Associate Professor
Division Coordinator, Athletic Training
Ohio University
Athens, OH

SECTION I

GENERAL INFORMATION

The Effective Approved Clinical Instructor

Thomas G. Weidner, PhD, ATC, FNATA

INTRODUCTION

So you have decided to serve as a clinical instructor. Maybe you want to invest in the development of young professionals who represent the future of the athletic training profession, or maybe you want to somehow give back to the profession for its importance in your life. Perhaps you are proud of your institution's athletic training education program, and you want to contribute. You may feel that working with athletic training students during their clinical education is refreshing and challenging, and compels you to stay abreast of the field. Now that you are committed to the clinical instructor role, you might as well do it well.

According to the accreditation standards from the Commission on the Accreditation of Athletic Training Education (CAATE), there are two different designations of clinical instructors who work with athletic training students.[1]

1. Approved Clinical Instructor (ACI):

   o Credentialed in a health care profession as defined by the American Medical Association or American Osteopathic Association (eg, physical therapist, physician assistant, EMT)

   o Identified and trained by the Athletic Training Education Program (ATEP) Clinical Instructor Educator (CIE) (see Chapter 7) to provide instruction and evaluation of the Athletic Training Education Competencies and/or Clinical Proficiencies.

   o The ACI may not be a current student within the ATEP.

2. Clinical Instructor (CI):

   o A credentialed health care professional as defined by the American Medical Association or the American Osteopathic Association

   o Identified to provide supervision of athletic training students during their clinical experiences.

o An ACI may be a CI, but all CIs do not have to be ACIs.

o If a CI credentialed for less than 1 year, the ATEP must develop and document the implementation of a plan for supervision of that CI by an experienced credentialed CI which ensures the quality of instruction provided to the athletic training students.

o A Clinical Instructor is not charged with the final formal evaluation of AT student's integration of clinical proficiencies (only an ACI can perform such evaluations).

Certainly, there is a great need for effective ACIs (and CIs), both for quality patient/athlete health care and for quality education of future athletic trainers. Effective clinical instruction fosters more competent practitioners. With the expanded responsibility you are taking on as an ACI, you will help shape athletic training students both professionally and personally. Athletic training students perceive that fully 53% of their professional development comes from clinical education.[2] By expanding your responsibilities to include those of an ACI, you will help shape not only the development of an athletic training student as a professional, but also as a person. Athletic training clinical education in general, and clinical instructors specifically, cannot simply and narrowly focus on athletic training students' skills and knowledge. This chapter is designed to help you to appreciate the roles and best practices of an ACI. Ways to manage role strain as the ACI who juggles responsibilities to students and patients will be briefly discussed as well. See Appendix A regarding online clinical teaching resources that are intended to augment this chapter.

SETTING IT RIGHT

Reflections regarding clinical education warrant attention.[3] Athletic trainers have a unique blend of abilities that are applied to the practice of athletic training. What is needed or valued at any time depends on the context—practical intervention, diagnostic expertise, or simply a caring attitude and understanding.[4] Borrowing from Harden et al,[5] there is a three-circle model (ie, inner, middle, and outer circles) that depicts these different abilities (Figure 1-1).

The inner circle, practical skills, represents the athletic trainer's knowledge, (eg, physical examination of a patient)—doing the right thing, taking the correct action. Interestingly, it can be equated with technical intelligence, in line with Gardner's multiple intelligences model.[6] The middle circle represents the way the athletic trainer approaches the tasks in the inner circle (ie, appropriate analytical strategies—in other words, doing the thing right). This includes the academic, analytical, and creative intelligences. The outer circle represents the development of the personal attributes of the individual (eg, ethics). In other words, the right person doing it. It equates with the personal and emotional intelligences. Particularly in this outer circle, some athletic trainers may excel, differentiating star performers from others. Professional expertise is more than mere baseline competence, and outstanding professionals usually have special personal attributes. You need to get the job and get it done, but how you do the job (ie, the other competencies you bring to your expertise) determines actual performance. Data from a number of studies suggest that, in general, emotional and personal competencies play a far larger role in superior job performance than do cognitive abilities and technical expertise.[7] Thus, one of your students may have all the technical competences in the inner circle, but still not be a good athletic trainer. The outcomes in the middle and outer circles mean that the student has to think as an athletic trainer.

Figure 1-1. Model depicting abilities of an athletic trainer.

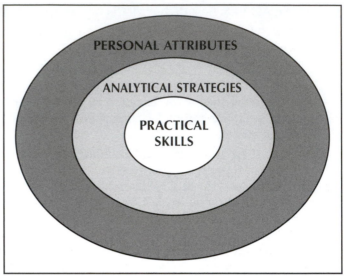

This three-circle model also acknowledges the need for a range of strategies and approaches to be an effective ACI. Drawing some parallels here, we cannot be all about teaching the right thing. Strategic approaches to learning, such as problem-based learning, can contribute to the achievement of the learning outcomes in the middle circle. In other words, teaching how to do the thing right. Role modeling can be important for the *achievement* of outcomes in the outer circle, thus teaching about the right person doing it.[5]

Perhaps we need to take on a servant attitude to our students through mentoring and role modeling. This likely will have more impact on our students as professionals than the content we actually teach. Effective ACIs are the backbone of the growth and development of our profession, and its professionals, as a whole. An ACI's success is measured by the success of students in the profession.

GETTING IT RIGHT

How do you get your role as an ACI right? How do you know that you are effective? How do you identify your specific strengths and weaknesses as an ACI?

Six standards and associated criteria for the effective ACI have been developed through research (Table 1-1).[8] These standards can be used as a point of reflection for your practices as an ACI, and to help you to develop a plan of action for the improvement of those practices. These standards and criteria can also serve as the foundation for the evaluation of your teaching practices by athletic training students and colleagues.

For these purposes, related CIE (Clinical Instructor Educator), self-evaluation, and student/peer evaluation forms have been developed to serve as models for the improvement of ACIs (see Appendices B through D).

These best-practice standards are considered universally important and applicable by certified athletic trainers in various clinical education settings (ie, colleges/universities, clinics, and high schools).[9] In particular, the legal and ethical behavior,

TABLE 1-1

STANDARDS FOR THE EFFECTIVE ATHLETIC TRAINING CLINICAL INSTRUCTOR

STANDARD	DESCRIPTION
Legal and Ethical Behavior	Comply with the NATA Code of Ethics and BOC Standards of Professional Practice.
Communication Skills	Communicate effectively with the Program Director and/or Clinical Education Coordinator and athletic training students.
Interpersonal Relationships	Enter into positive and effective interpersonal relationships with students, including being a role model and mentor.
Instructional Skills	Demonstrate effective instructional skills during clinical education, including a basic knowledge of educational principles.
Supervisory and Administrative Skills	Provide the right type, amount, and quality of clinical supervision and uphold the clinical education policies, procedures, and expectations of the Athletic Training Education Program.
Evaluation of Performance	Inform students of the strengths and weaknesses of their clinical performance.
Clinical Skills and Knowledge	Demonstrate appropriate clinical competence in the field of athletic training through sound evidence-based practice and clinical decision-making.

communication skills, interpersonal relationships, and clinical skills and knowledge standards are considered the most important, applicable, and crucial. Legal and ethical behavior was considered the most crucial standard. The large majority (92%) of the respondents in the research to develop these standards and related forms[9] reported that unsatisfactory legal and ethical behavior would justify eliminating the ACI from the clinical education program. However, the respondents do indicate that there are practical barriers (eg, role strain, time demands) in the full use of the standards (see section below for additional comments).

THE RIGHT STANDARDS

What follows is a presentation of the six standards/criteria and their application to ACIs and clinical education. Although the focus is on the ACI, it is understood that the Director of the Athletic Training Education Program and/or coordinator of clinical education also have critical roles and responsibilities in effectively implementing these standards.

Legal and Ethical Behavior

For certified athletic trainers, legal and ethical behavior includes abiding by the NATA Code of Ethics[10] and the BOC Standards of Professional Practice,[11] which are designed to keep athletic trainers aware of the professional conduct required in the practice of athletic training. The Code represents ethical principles and standards for all certified athletic trainers. Of particular importance to ACIs is compliance with federal, state, and local laws and regulations governing the practice of the profession. Examples include equal opportunity and affirmative action policies, Americans with Disabilities Act (ADA), Health Insurance Portability and Accountability Act (HIPAA), and Family Educational Rights and Privacy Act (FERPA). Regarding the athletic training profession, most states have a form of regulation (ie, registration, certification, licensure, and exemption), that will affect the roles of certified athletic trainers as ACIs.[12] Also, the BOC (Board of Certification) requires all certified athletic trainers to obtain 75 continuing education units every 3 years in order to maintain certification status.[13] Individuals who do not fulfill the continuing education requirements are placed on probation. Certainly, any irresponsible behavior regarding state regulation or BOC certification would provide a poor professional example for athletic training students.

Communication Skills

ACIs need to communicate regularly (ie, at scheduled intervals) with the Program Director and/or Clinical Education Coordinator regarding athletic training student progress towards clinical education goals determined by the ATEP. This would include using appropriate forms of communication to clearly and concisely express yourself to athletic training students, both verbally and in writing. Appropriately timed and constructive formative and summative feedback to athletic training students is also essential in this communication (see Chapter 12).

Also, frequently communicate with athletic training students through open-ended questions and directed problem solving. Set time aside to ensure ongoing professional discussions with your athletic training students, setting a nonconfrontational and positive tone.

Several studies indicate that effective communication skills are essential for a successful teaching/learning exchange to occur.[14-18] The effective ACI must draw on a broad range of communication skills to choose the most appropriate communication style for the teaching situation.[19] Your communication style should be nonthreatening to students.[15-17] Along these same lines, ACIs must recognize the importance of correcting students tactfully while providing a clear, honest perception of the student's abilities.[17,18]

You would also do well to engage in positive communication behaviors that encourage student-teacher dialogue. For instance, demonstrate active listening skills and ask open-ended questions to create an environment that illustrates sincere interest.[14,17,18] Try to clearly explain clinical problems and expectations in a comprehensible manner,[17] maintaining a balance between sharing information and permitting freedom of discussion.[18]

Interpersonal Relationships

As an ACI, try to enter into positive and effective interpersonal relationships with your students. This would include being a role model and mentor.[18,20,21] Because interpersonal relationships are crucial in making the student feel valued as a person,[18] ACIs should approach the teaching/learning process and student interaction with enthusiasm and positivism.[18,20,22-24] You should not only be friendly, honest, and approachable but should also show a genuine interest and concern for the student as a learner and as a person.[15,16,18,22,25] Basically, the approach here needs to be how can I help you, not how can you help me. Further, ACIs need to model appropriate and professional interpersonal relationships when interacting with other athletic training students, colleagues, patients/athletes, and administrators. Try to be an advocate for your athletic training students when interacting with these individuals. Certainly, ACIs should demonstrate respect for gender, racial, ethnic, religious, and individual differences when interacting with people. Moreover, because the clinical setting is distinct from the classroom in that it includes patient care,[26] it is essential that you set an example of sincere interest in your patients, as well as in your students.[2,16,18,27] Also, through self-disclosure you can relate to your students that they are not alone in the learning process and that certain deficiencies, stresses, and frustrations are common during clinical practice and education in the clinical environment.[28]

Through effective interpersonal relationships, ACIs can foster and encourage professional behavior in their students at all times.

Instructional Skills

The ACI needs to demonstrate effective instructional skills during the clinical education experience, including a basic knowledge of educational principles regarding clinical teaching[29] (see Chapters 4 and 5). There is a connection between clinical education and the principles of adult education,[30] and students involved in the clinical education component of athletic training education should be viewed as adults who are voluntarily pursuing the profession. Help your students both formally and informally, utilizing teachable moments wherever they occur. You will want to implement and evaluate planned learning experiences as well as take advantage of unplanned opportunities that occur during clinical practice. Instruct and practice meaningful skills or content with your students, and apply immediately if possible. To be most effective, you will need to understand your athletic training students' academic curriculum, level of didactic preparation, and current level of performance, relative to the goals of the clinical education experience. This may then likely include modifying your students' learning experiences based on their strengths and weaknesses. The ACI needs to be able to communicate complicated/detailed concepts in terms that students can understand based on their level of progression within the athletic training education program. In order to meet the needs of different learners, employ a variety of teaching styles (see Chapter 5). The ACI needs to ultimately create learning opportunities that actively engage their athletic training students in the clinical setting and that promote problem-solving and critical thinking. So that students do not become overly dependent on your assistance, the ACI should encourage self-directed learning activities for the athletic training students when appropriate. You would do well to encourage your athletic training students to engage in self-directed learning as a means of establishing life-long learning practices of inquiry and clinical problem solving. However, also try to foster a spirit of collaboration among your students through peer teaching/learning and clinical problem solving[15,17,31,32] (see Chapter 8). In order to develop connections between theoretical content taught in the classroom and practical clinical applications, create opportunities for critical reflection among your students as a planned feature of your clinical education (eg, student logs or update reports).[15-18]

Ultimately, the ACI needs to be enthusiastic about teaching athletic training students and should perform regular self-appraisal of his/her teaching methods and effectiveness (see Appendix C).

Supervisory and Administrative Skills

The ACI needs effective supervisory skills in the clinical setting. In accordance with CAATE Standards,[1] the ACIs must directly supervise athletic training students during formal acquisition, practice, and evaluation of the Entry-Level Athletic Training Clinical Proficiencies. The ACI must be able to intervene on behalf of the athlete/patient when the athletic training student is putting the athlete/patient at risk or harm.[1] When appropriate, encourage athletic training students to arrive at clinical decisions on their own, according to their level of education and clinical experience. However, treat the athletic training students' presence as educational and not as a means for providing service or medical coverage.

Also, establish a positive environment for the teaching/learning exchange to occur.[16,17,24] In certain situations (eg, side line evaluation of a knee injury), this may include encouraging and providing extra supervision when new and/or difficult clinical situations arise, remaining readily accessible, and serving as a resource for students.[15-18] However, maintain a balance between providing too much supervision and fostering student autonomy.[20,21] You will need to make a decision, based on the knowledge and experience level of the student, when to withhold supervision in order to promote confidence and growth in your students' clinical skills (see Chapters 3 and 9).

Effective ACIs will also need strong administrative skills, as many ACIs have responsibilities within the athletics department as well as within an academic department. Therefore, ACIs must be able to manage time and to delegate tasks.[17] There are various administrative inter-relationships between the ACI, student, setting, and academic program that require attention. The ACI will need to uphold the clinical education policies, procedures, and expectations of the Athletic Training Education Program. Potential administrative tasks associated with clinical education include completing clinical performance evaluation forms for students and documenting their clinical progression in completing the required clinical proficiencies. ACIs also need to conduct productive and timely conferences regarding student performance.[18] ACIs will also need to inform their athletic training students of relevant policies and procedures of their particular clinical setting.

Evaluation of Performance

In order to teach students appropriate patient care, ACIs must effectively evaluate and assess students' skills, as in any allied health care profession.[32] Without appropriate evaluation, mistakes go uncorrected, good performance is not reinforced, and clinical competence is compromised.[32] Evaluation assists the student in attaining entry-level competence by informing the student of his/her current level of performance, and by identifying strengths and weaknesses compared to specified standards.[33] Provide feedback to your athletic training students from information acquired from your direct observation, discussion with others, and review of athlete/patient documentation. This provides you with the information necessary to design further quality learning experiences and to modify existing ones. Additionally, evaluation provides academic and clinical information regarding student progress, enabling ACIs to assign student grades, to determine whether students have attained entry-level competence, and to assess the effectiveness of the academic and clinical curricula.[34]

The overriding consideration in clinical evaluation is whether or not the student's level of clinical performance is acceptable. Note your athletic training students' knowledge, skills, and behaviors as they relate to the specific goals and objectives of their clinical experience, identifying areas of competence as well as areas that require improvement. The ACI needs to approach this evaluation process as constructive and educational, using both formative (ie, on going specific feedback) and summative (ie, general overall performance feedback) assessment (see Chapter 12). If an athletic training student needs remediation, communicate with the Program Director and/or Coordinator of Clinical Education in a timely manner.

Clinical Skills and Knowledge

ACIs should demonstrate appropriate clinical competence in the field of athletic training through sound clinical decision-making[24] and a systematic approach to problem solving.[17] Explain to your students the basis for your actions and clinical decisions.[16] Your clinical knowledge and skills must be current and your care decisions based on science and evidence-based practice. It is also imperative that the ACI be able to demonstrate the appropriate role of the athletic trainer within the total health care team.[17]

Certainly by virtue of holding and maintaining the ATC credential, any certified athletic trainer is clinically competent as measured by the BOC *Role Delineation Study: Athletic Training Profession*. However, further competence is desired in the 12 educational content areas of athletic training indicated in the NATA *Athletic Training Educational Competencies*[35]:

1. Risk Management and Injury Prevention
2. Pathology of Injuries and Illnesses
3. Orthopedic Clinical Examination and Diagnosis
4. Medical Conditions and Disabilities
5. Acute Care of Injuries and Illnesses
6. Therapeutic Modalities
7. Conditioning and Rehabilitative Exercise
8. Pharmacology
9. Psychosocial Intervention and Referral
10. Nutritional Aspects of Injuries and Illnesses
11. Health Care Administration
12. Professional Development and Responsibility

THE RIGHT BALANCE

Clinical educators often experience role strain as they attempt to balance roles in clinical education with roles in patient care.[9] Goode's[36] long-standing role theory provides a framework for understanding the role strain experienced by ACIs, suggesting that in general, people want to fulfill all of the expectations placed upon them. However, there will certainly be some cases in which they are unable to do so. To further appreciate this theory and its relevance to role strain experienced by ACIs, it is necessary to define key operational terms.

First, a *role occupant* is an individual occupying a particular role. For example, an athletic trainer (AT) may occupy the role of an ACI, health care provider, or administrator. Often times, however, the athletic trainer is simultaneously occupying these roles. A *role set* comprises a group of relationships associated with occupying a particular role. For example, the ACI role set may include relationships with athletic training students, the program director, and the clinical education coordinator. As a health care provider, the role set may include relationships with patients, physicians, and coaches. As an administrator, the role set may include relationships with athletic directors and insurance coordinators. *Role obligations* are those expectations associated with occupying a particular role and are defined by the members of the role set. The athletic trainer, then, has expectations from the individuals in each of the role sets mentioned above. For example, program directors expect athletic trainers as ACIs to complete required student evaluations in a timely manner. Patients expect the athletic trainer, as a health care provider, to render high quality care that will enable them to return to competition as quickly as possible. Athletic directors expect the athletic trainer as administrator to monitor supply budgets and keep costs low. *Role strain*, then, is manifested when an individual has difficulty meeting the various obligations associated with the multiple roles.[36] Therefore, according to Goode's[36] role theory, an athletic trainer who simultaneously occupies the roles of ACI, health care provider, and administrator may not be able to fulfill all of the role expectations (eg, expectations from the program director, athletic director, etc). Conflicts associated with time commitments and priorities may arise and may result in role strain.[37]

One strategy to reduce role strain is to eliminate the number of role relationships, particularly those about which you may have less interest and/or about which you feel incompetent. For instance, graduate assistant athletic trainers often accept a position to enhance clinical experience, not necessarily to serve as ACIs. A new professional may find it difficult to take on the additional role of ACI due to an already overwhelming role set as clinician and graduate student. In a perfect world, these fledgling athletic trainers would not be expected to provide clinical instruction. However, because many ATEPs rely on graduate assistant athletic trainers (who have a minimum of 1 year of clinical experience) to serve as ACIs, steps should be taken to ensure that they are receiving adequate orientation for this role. Therefore, it may benefit ATEPs to gradually introduce graduate assistant athletic trainers to the ACI role during the first year, progressively leading up to serve as ACIs during the second year.

Other steps may reduce role strain. ATEP administrators could provide ACIs with a clinical education handbook that outlines the ATEP's curriculum, clinical education policies, evaluation tools, and expectations of the ACI.[38] Also, ATEP administrators should be sensitive to time demands on ACIs and flexible in student clinical assignments. ACIs may occasionally need a break from supervising students.[38] Further, ATEPs may consider assigning athletic training students with the same academic level (eg, junior students) to an ACI each rotation so that the ACI can develop consistency in expectations and efficiency in assessments.[38,39] For example, an ACI who is simultaneously supervising three different levels of students is juggling three different sets of performance expectations and three different evaluation tools.

ACIs in an ATEP with a positive climate will experience less role strain. This could be fostered through ACI accessibility to the CIE[40] and through open communication between program administrators, ACIs, and students.[41]

REFLECTION QUESTIONS

Draw your own insights about whether you may be an effective Approved Clinical Instructor by answering these questions:

- Why are you interested in becoming, or continuing to be, an ACI?
- Do you distinguish between doing the right thing, doing the thing right, and the right person doing it?
- Do you utilize best practice standards for becoming an effective ACI?
- Do you recognize the sources of your role strain and take actions to modify them?

REFERENCES

1. Commission on Accreditation of Athletic Training Education. Standards for the accreditation of entry-level athletic training education programs. August 8, 2007; http://caate.net/ss_docs/standards.6.8.2006.pdf. Accessed November 7, 2007.
2. Laurent T, Weidner TG. Clinical Instructors' and student athletic trainers' perceptions of helpful Clinical Instructor characteristics. *J Athl Train*. 2001;36(1):58-61.
3. Weidner TG. Reflection on athletic training education reform. *Athl Train Educ J*. 2006;1(1):6-7.
4. Harden RM, Davis MH, Crosby JR. The new Dundee medical curriculum: a whole that is greater than the sum of the parts. *Med Educ*. 1997;31(4):264-271.
5. Harden RM, Crosby JR. Outcome-based education: Part 5-From competence to meta-competency. *Med Teach*. 1999;2:546.
6. Gardner H. *Frames of Mind*. New York: Basic Books; 1983.
7. Goleman D. *Working with Emotional Intelligence*. Vol 21. London: Bloomsbury; 1998.
8. Weidner TG, Henning JM. Development of standards and criteria for the selection, training, and evaluation of athletic training approved Clinical Instructors. *J Athl Train*. 2004;39(4):335-343.
9. Weidner TG, Henning JM. Importance and applicability of approved Clinical Instructor standards and criteria to certified athletic trainers in different clinical education settings. *J Athl Train*. 2005;40(4):326-332.
10. National Athletic Trainers' Association. Code of Ethics. Available at: http://www.nata.org/codeofethics/code_of_ethics.pdf. Accessed November 7, 2007.
11. Board of Certification. BOC Standards of Professional Practice. November 6, 2007; Available at: http://www.bocatc.org/images/stories/multiple_references/standardsprofessionalpractice.pdf. Accessed November 14, 2007.
12. Ray R. *Management Strategies in Athletic Training*. 2nd ed. Champaign, IL: Human Kinetics; 2000:220-237.
13. Board of Certification. Recertification Requirements (2006-2011). November 6, 2007; Available at: http://www.bocatc.org/images/stories/athletic_trainers/recertificationrequirements2006-2011.pdf. Accessed November 14, 2007.
14. Weidner TG, Trethewey J. Learning clinical skills in athletic training. *Athl Ther Today*. 1997;2(5):43-49.
15. Jarski RW, Kulig K, Olson RE. Clinical teaching in physical therapy: student and teacher perceptions. *Phys Ther*. 1990;70(3):173-178.
16. Gjerde CL, Coble RJ. Resident and faculty perceptions of effective clinical teaching in family practice. *J Fam Pract*. 1982;14(2):323-327.
17. Emery MJ. Effectiveness of the Clinical Instructor. Students' perspective. *Phys Ther*. 1984;64(7):1079-1083.
18. Dunlevy CL, Wolf KN. Perceived differences in the importance and frequency of practice of clinical teaching behaviors. *J Allied Health*. 1992;21(3):175-183.
19. Schwenk TL. *Clinical Teaching*. New York: Center for Research on Learning and Teaching; 1987.
20. Irby DM, Ramsey PG, Gillmore GM, Schaad D. Characteristics of effective clinical teachers of ambulatory care medicine. *Acad Med*. 1991;66(1):54-55.
21. Andersen MB, Larson GA, Luebe JJ. Student and Supervisor Perceptions of the Quality of Supervision in Athletic Training Education. *J Athl Train*. 1997;32(4):328-332.

22. Nehring V. Nursing clinical teacher effectiveness inventory: A replication study of the characteristics of 'best' and 'worst' clinical teachers as perceived by nursing faculty and students. *J Adv Nurs.* 1990;15(8):934-940.

23. Knox JE, Mogan J. Important clinical teacher behaviours as perceived by university nursing faculty, students and graduates. *J Adv Nurs.* 1985;10(1):25-30.

24. Curtis N, Helion JG, Domsohn M. Student Athletic Trainer Perceptions of Clinical Supervisor Behaviors: A Critical Incident Study. *J Athl Train.* 1998;33(3):249-253.

25. Mogan J, Knox JE. Characteristics of the 'best' and 'worst' clinical teachers as perceived by university nursing faculty and students. *J Adv Nurs.* 1987;12:331-337.

26. Weidner TG, Henning JM. Being an effective athletic training Clinical Instructor. *Athl Ther Today.* 2002;7(5):6-11.

27. *NATA Education Council Newsletter.* 2001;3:3.

28. Bauer LC, Alexander A. Skills in clinical teaching: a faculty development program for resident optometrists. *J Optomet Educ.* 1984;9:16-19.

29. Deusinger SS, Cornbleet SL, Stith JS. Using assessment centers to promote clinical faculty development. *J Phys Ther Educ.* 1991;5:14-17.

30. McGaghie WC, Stritter FT. Principles of clinical education. *Alcohol Health Res World.* 1989;13(1):28-31.

31. Triggs-Nemshick M, Shepard KF. Physical therapy clinical education in a 2:1 student-instructor education model. *Phys Ther.* 1996;76:968-981.

32. Ende J. Feedback in clinical medical education. *Jama.* 1983;250(6):777-781.

33. Weidner TG, August JA, Welles R, Pelletier D. Evaluating clinical skills in athletic therapy. *Athl Ther Today.* 1998;3(3):26-30.

34. Campbell SK. Development of psychomotor objectives for classroom or clinical education in physical therapy. *Phys Ther.* 1977;57(9):1031-1034.

35. National Athletic Trainers' Association. *Athletic Training Educational Competencies.* 4th ed. Dallas, TX: National Athletic Trainers' Association; 2006.

36. Goode WJ. A theory of role strain. *Amer Soc Rev.* 1960;25(4):483-496.

37. Henning JM, Weidner TG. Collegiate athletic training approved Clinical Instructors are experiencing role strain. *J Athl Train.* 2008;43 (3):275-283.

38. Hildebrandt E. Preceptors: a perspective of what works. *Clin Excell Nurse Pract.* 2001;5(3):175-180.

39. Oermann MH. Role strain of clinical nursing faculty. *J Prof Nurs.* 1998;14(6):329-334: 275-283.

40. Langan JC. Faculty practice and roles of staff nurses and clinical faculty in nursing student learning. *J Prof Nurs.* 2003;19(2):76-84.

41. Piscopo B. Organizational climate, communication, and role strain in clinical nursing faculty. *J Prof Nurs.* 1994; 10(2):113-119.

2

The Coordination and Delivery of Athletic Training Clinical Education

Thomas G. Weidner, PhD, ATC, FNATA

Athletic training clinical education seeks to teach students to apply the knowledge and skills they have learned in classrooms and laboratories to actual practice on patients, under supervision of an approved clinical instructor (ACI)/clinical instructor (CI).[1] integrating the theoretical and practical educational components from the classroom and laboratory into real-life situations with actual athletes or patients.[2] Such experiences are vital to a student's development of competence, self-confidence, and flexibility in new, unfamiliar situations.[3] As few limitations are placed on which activities constitute clinical education, the hands-on activities can include any experience that provides a practical or applied focus. For instance, students might practice their psychomotor skills in a simulated environment on simulated patients. Clinical education progresses from specific technical skills to clinical competence with actual patients.[4] Also during clinical education, students must learn to be professionals.[5] Clinical education, a triad involving the interplay between setting, instructor, and student, constitutes a substantial portion of professional preparation in the allied health care fields. Entry-level certified athletic trainers perceive that approximately 53% of their entry-level professional development came from clinical education.[6]

The purpose of this chapter is to help you to better coordinate and deliver clinical education in your setting. This will first include understanding the important similarities and differences between academic and clinical instruction. Eliminating randomness in your students' clinical experiences, effective communicating among the clinical education team, and developing and evaluating your clinical education setting for delivering clinical education will then be discussed.

ACADEMIC VERSUS CLINICAL INSTRUCTION

Clinical instruction cannot be separated from academic (classroom) instruction as though they are two distinct entities. Educational programs are designed to incorporate the clinical education component in one of two patterns. In the concurrent pattern, the student is simultaneously completing academic and clinical education. Ideal clinical experiences are those that are closely relevant and timely to what is being taught in concurrent courses and that allow continued reinforcement and practice of what has been learned. In the nonconcurrent pattern, the student completes the clinical education on a full-time basis upon completion of the academic program (or at a defined phase of the academic program). Academic instruction in the classroom/lab and clinical instruction in the clinical setting have several similarities, but their differences are significant. The differences center on the nature of the learning experience, teaching methods, and professional/social relationship of the student to the faculty.

Learning in academic education often occurs in a predictable classroom environment that is characterized by a beginning and ending of the learning session. The subject matter is usually detailed. Academic instruction can be presented in many formats with varying degrees of structure (eg, lecture formats with the use of audiovisuals, laboratory practice, problem-based case discussions, independent online learning, or group work).[7] Learning objectives in the classroom are commonly based in the cognitive domain, emphasizing knowledge, understanding, synthesis, and evaluation. They foster the ability to solve problems on a theoretical basis. Fundamental concepts and theories, and their practical application in the athletic training profession, are developed as the student progresses through the academic program.[8] Further, clinical skills are learned and practiced in simulated environments. There is more of a social distance between the classroom instructor and the student during academic instruction. Teachers and students can hide their personalities in the typically more rigid classroom environment through lower levels of participation and interaction.

In contrast, clinical instruction is more dynamic and flexible. This is because the clinical environment is far more unpredictable. Learning objectives in clinical education emphasize practical skills, clinical judgment, and communication skills. Clinical instruction and practice are less structured. As well, student learning is usually not measured by written examinations, but by the quality, efficiency, and outcomes of the student's patient care. In contrast to academic instruction, personalities are hard to suppress and are usually evident in the beginning of the clinical experience. The nature of the clinical environment fosters close social interaction among the Approved Clinical Instructor (ACI), the student, and the patient. Therefore, students certainly tend to learn some of their roles by simply observing ACIs providing patient care. Thus, our students' professional behaviors begin to reflect more and more those of their ACIs.[8] These modeled behaviors influence the student's lifetime professional performance.[9,10] It is safe to assume that ACIs influence the student's future professional style and demeanor considerably more than academic instructors. This turns out to be quite a responsibility.

ELIMINATE RANDOMNESS

Although athletic training students learn some of their professional responsibilities by simply observing and modeling ACIS, formal and consistent clinical education helps to ensure that all students are exposed to a comprehensive, uniform clinical experience during their professional preparation.

A lack of formal emphasis on clinical instruction promotes haphazard and coincidental learning during students' clinical experiences. Instruction may not be consistent from one clinical experience to the next or from one ACI to the next. Such disorder may occur because many clinicians have not been taught to teach in the clinical setting. Often, ACIs have only their own student background to direct them in their methods and strategies regarding clinical instruction. ACIs tend to focus more closely on the patient/athlete than on the athletic training student as well. Effective clinical instruction, however, applies a thoughtful and proactive approach to teaching clinical skills.

Today's ACIs are responsible for initiating educational opportunities for their students in the clinical setting. Although patient/athlete safety is still of utmost importance, the focus in clinical instruction must include educational experiences designed to augment your students' knowledge and to promote their professional maturity. Clinical instruction progresses from knowledge and skill competencies (ie, competency-based clinical education) to clinical proficiencies. The 4th edition of the *Athletic Training Educational Competencies* (ATEC) contains the clinical competencies and proficiencies for effective preparation of the entry-level athletic trainer.[5] These clinical competencies/proficiencies are organized into 12 content areas, around which athletic training courses are organized. Competencies are specific, professional, entry-level knowledge and skills that students should be able to demonstrate upon completion of the athletic training education program (eg, knee injury stress tests). In contrast, the clinical proficiencies guide decision making and skill integration (eg, knee injury evaluation).[5] Thus, the proficiencies are "real-life" applications of the specific knowledge and skill competencies.[11] Foundational behaviors of professional practice intertwine with the application of clinical competencies/proficiencies in working with real patients, including primacy of the patient, legal practice, ethical practice, cultural competence, and professionalism (see Appendix E).

Ultimately, ACIs should develop learning objectives for each clinical education rotation to reflect appropriate clinical competencies/proficiencies and foundations of professional practice for students at a particular level (eg, beginning, intermediate, advanced). It is the ACI's job to implement, and then evaluate, these objectives into the individual athletic training student's clinical experiences. These objectives coincide with the learning objectives in the concurrent courses being completed by the athletic training student.

EFFECTIVE COMMUNICATION

Successfully integrating classroom knowledge into clinical practice requires a team effort, including the program director, academic faculty, ACIs, coordinator of clinical education, setting coordinator of clinical education, and students. Communication among these various individuals is vitally important to the education process.[12,13] The more people involved with communication, however, the greater the chance for misunderstanding.[14,15] Specific learning objectives for clinical experiences and frequent interactions among all team members should help to keep communication clear.

Often the program director or another athletic training faculty member at each institution serves as the coordinator of clinical education. The duties of the coordinator of clinical education could include developing, implementing, and evaluating athletic training clinical education experiences. As ATEPs utilize additional clinical experience settings, a single coordinator of clinical education likely becomes more important.

Medicine[16] and physical therapy[17] also suggest using a coordinator of clinical education at each clinical setting. Duties would include coordinating clinical experiences in accordance with the clinical education objectives determined by the ATEP and communicated through the coordinator of clinical education. The staff member appointed as the setting coordinator of clinical education needs to be proficient as a clinician, experienced in clinical education, and interested in students. Further, this person needs to have good interpersonal relationship and organizational skills and be knowl-edgeable of the facility and its resources. The setting coordinator keeps the channels of communication open among students, other ACIs at the setting, ATEP administra-tors, and the coordinator of clinical education. In this way, there will be less chance for miscommunication and confusion.

Research has revealed, however, that the more complex the clinical education structure, the lower the students will rate the educational experiences.[18] Hopefully, the coordinator of clinical education and the setting coordinator of clinical education should be able to minimize the confusion that may occur when multiple students are involved with many clinical instructors. Ultimately, the lubrication for coordinating and delivering effective clinical education requires a close and productive relationship between the coordinator of clinical education and the setting coordinator of clinical education at each clinical site. Further, regular and frequent meetings among the clini-cal education team to communicate about a variety of educational issues and to build camaraderie among the team is highly desirable. Students benefit when they sense unity among the team.

DEVELOPING THE CLINICAL SETTING FOR DELIVERING CLINICAL EDUCATION

Clinical education settings must include educational standards and experiences designed to augment students' knowledge and to promote their professional compe-tence. There are a variety of essential personnel, administrative, and environmental factors involved in high-quality clinical education settings.[4] Basically, we cannot expect to prepare high-quality athletic training professionals in poor or questionable clinical education settings. Simply spending time in clinical experiences does not ensure that students acquire adequate clinical skills.[4] Unfortunately, there are times when structured learning experiences are not even possible at some of our clinical education settings. If you think about it, more often than not, settings are selected somewhat at random for convenience, geographical location, and availability of "slots" for students.[4] However, as slightly over half of athletic training professional develop-ment was perceived by entry-level certified athletic trainers to come from clinical education,[6] clinical settings will need to be structured, developed, and evaluated to ensure that optimal education is taking place. Again, failure to objectively develop and evaluate the settings may result in chance learning. Such learning is contrary to the purpose and requirements of accreditation, especially regarding the quality of athletic training clinical education.[1] Let us acknowledge here that we cannot expect to provide comprehensive clinical education solely in the traditional athletic training room. Clinical education is expected in a variety of medical and health care settings. However, no matter the specific setting (ie, traditional athletic training room or allied medical), there are a number of factors or standards (in addition to effective commu-nications and coordinators of clinical education mentioned above) that should be con-sidered in developing a high-quality clinical education setting (Table 2-1).[4] Especially note how these factors are student centered.

Learning Environment

An effective clinical setting will have good management, high staff morale, harmo-nious working relationships, and sound interdisciplinary patient management proce-

TABLE 2-1

ESSENTIAL PERSONNEL, ADMINISTRATIVE, AND ENVIRONMENTAL FACTORS INVOLVED IN COORDINATING AND DELIVERING CLINICAL EDUCATION

- The clinical education setting provides an active, stimulating environment appropriate for the learning needs of the student. (Learning environment)

- Clinical education programs for students are planned to meet specific objectives of the educational program and the individual student. (Learning objectives)

- The clinical education setting has a variety of learning experiences available to students. (Learning experiences)

- The clinical education setting demonstrates administrative interest in and support of athletic training clinical education. (Administrative support)

- Communications within the clinical education setting are effective and positive. (Effective communications)

- The clinical instructors are adequate in number to provide a good educational program for students. (Staff number)

- One clinical instructor with specific qualifications is responsible for coordinating the assignments and activities of the students at the clinical setting. (Setting coordinator of clinical education)

- Adequate space for study, conference, and treating athletes/patients is available to students. (Adequate space)

Reprinted with permission from Laurent T, Weidner TG. Clinical-education-setting standards are helpful in the professional preparation of employed, entry-level certified athletic trainers. *J Athl Train*. 2002;37(4 Suppl):S248-S254.

dures. Further, a desirable learning experience requires that health care personnel are receptive to students, have varied areas of expertise, are interested in new techniques, and are involved with professions outside athletic training.

Learning Objectives

Successful clinical education experiences need specific learning objectives. The use of learning objectives is a commonly accepted practice in pedagogy and should be central to planning clinical education experiences. Objectives improve the uniformity of the educational experience, providing a framework for both students and ACIs. For example, developing student update reports centered around specific clinical education objectives can create uniformity. Students could provide summary comments regarding their global experiences (eg, general quality of experience, general satisfaction with experience) and their local experiences (eg, experiences regarding specific target objectives, such as lower extremity assessments during the semester in which that material is being learned).

Learning Experiences

Varied learning experiences are important not only because they provide more opportunities for students to learn but also because they provide students with a wider array of treatment options for their future professional use. These treatment options are often referred to as "tools in the toolbox." Because not every patient responds the same way to every treatment, professionals need to possess the knowledge and skill to address similar problems in a variety of ways and with a variety of patients.

Staff Number

Commission on Accreditation of Athletic Training Education (CAATE) standards[1] recommend a maximum of 8 students to 1 clinical instructor for appropriate overall clinical supervision. Ultimately, there needs to be a balance between students' quality clinical experiences and appropriate supervision. As well, supervision requires that a clinical instructor be close enough to intervene on behalf of the patient, if necessary. Sometimes a direct supervision ratio of 1 student to 1 clinical instructor would be best, for example, with inexperienced students. In contrast, experienced students need more autonomy and may benefit more from a larger student-to-clinical instructor ratio (eg, 8:1). All students require supervision, and the numbers should reflect that need, always leaving room for communication between the student and ACI.

Adequate Space

Proper environments for studying, conferencing, and treating athletes/patients would be helpful in clinical education. Research does demonstrate that facility design affects learning and can stimulate or stifle collaborative learning. As clinical sites are developed, ACIs need to be aware of the influence of physical facilities on learning.

Administrative Support

Considering the variety of roles and responsibilities of certified athletic trainers, it is not surprising that they may not have ample time to adequately serve as ACIs. The general trend is toward increased work loads to provide medical care coverage for expanding sport seasons and off-season conditioning, practice, and competition schedules—with fewer resources and pressures from all sides. A greater responsibility for the teaching, supervising, and assessing of students may often be unrealistic. Similar to what has occurred in nursing, ACIs may encounter role strain when there is conflict between the needs of the athlete/patient and the needs of the student.[19] In this situation, accountability to the patient will take precedence, as athletic training students cannot be a labor force to provide athletic medical care. Due to time constraints, ATEP administrators should take care to acknowledge the time it takes the clinical instructor to teach and evaluate clinical skills.

EVALUATION OF CLINICAL EDUCATION SETTINGS

In order to effectively develop any clinical education setting (traditional athletic training room or allied medical), it is important to identify strengths and weaknesses. With this information, the setting coordinator of clinical education, ACIs, and ATEP administrators can work together to address deficiencies. Developing and improving the quality of clinical education delivered in a particular clinical education setting will be an on-going effort. Clinical Education Setting Self-Assessment and Clinical Education Setting Student Assessment Forms[4] (see Appendix F) have been developed for that purpose, and are structured around the essential personnel, administrative, and environmental factors involved in high-quality clinical education settings presented above. Perhaps you would do well to have your students complete the student assessment form at the end of a clinical assignment (including intercollegiate athletic training room). The form could be submitted to the coordinator of clinical education for review and then forwarded to the setting coordinator of clinical education and ACIs. With input from all involved, ways to improve the setting can be discussed. A rubric for recognizing key deficiencies and specific plans to address these deficiencies for a given year has also been developed to facilitate this process (see Appendix G).

REFLECTION QUESTIONS

Draw your own insights about whether your clinical education setting is coordinating and delivering effective clinical education by answering these questions:

- Is there a true appreciation in your setting regarding the impact that ACIs have on students' professional development?

- Does your setting proactively implement strategies to eliminate randomness in students' clinical experiences?

- Are communications among your clinical education team organized and effective?

- Do you use standards for the development and evaluation of your clinical education setting?

REFERENCES

1. Commission on Accreditation of Athletic Training Education. Standards for the accreditation of entry-level athletic training education programs. Retrieved November 7, 2007, from http://caate.net/ss_docs/standards.6.8.2006.pdf .
2. Jarski RW, Kulig K, Olson RE. Clinical teaching in physical therapy: student and teacher perceptions. *Phys Ther.* 1990;70(3):173-178.
3. DeTornyay R. *Strategies for Teaching Nursing.* New York: John Wiley & Sons; 1987.
4. Weidner TG, Laurent T. Selection and evaluation guidelines for clinical education settings in athletic training. *J Athl Train.* 2001;36(1):62-67.
5. National Athletic Trainers' Association. *Athletic Training Educational Competencies.* 4th ed. Dallas, TX: Author; 2006.
6. Laurent T, Weidner TG. Clinical-education-setting standards are helpful in the professional preparation of employed, entry-level certified athletic trainers. *J Athl Train.* 2002;37(4 Suppl):S248-S254.
7. Brookfield S. *Self-directed Learning: From Theory to Practice.* Vol 25. San Francisco, CA: Jossey-Bass; 1985.
8. Gandy J. Preparation for teaching in clinical settings. In: Shepard KF, Jensen GM, eds. *Handbook for the Physical Therapist.* Boston, MA: Butterworth-Heinemann; 1977:122-126.
9. American Physical Therapy Association. *Clinical education guidelines and self-assessment.* Alexandria, VA: American Physical Therapy Association; 1993.
10. Commission of Accreditation in Physical Therapy Education. *Evaluation Criteria for Accreditation of Education Programs for the Preparation of Physical Therapists.* Alexandria, VA: American Physical Therapy Association; 1992.
11. Walker SE, Weidner TG, Armstrong KJ. Athletic training students' clinical proficiencies are primarily evaluated via simulations. *J Athl Train.* In press.

12. Emery MJ. Effectiveness of the clinical instructor: students' perspective. *Phys Ther.* 1984;64(7):1079-1083.
13. Swann E, Walker SE. Interpersonal communications of the athletic training clinical instructor. *J Athl Train.* 2001;36(suppl):S-48.
14. Hanson EM. *Educational Administration and Organizational Behavior.* 4th ed. Boston, MA: Allyn and Bacon; 1996.
15. Kowalski TJ. *The School Superintendent: Theory, Practice, and Cases.* Columbus, OH: Merrill Prentice Hall; 1999.
16. Anderson DC, Harris IB, Allen S, et al. Comparing students' feedback about clinical instruction with their performance. *Acad Med.* 1991;66:29-34.
17. American Physical Therapy Association. PT/PTA educators and clinical educators-information. Retrieved October 4, 2001, from: https://www.apta.org/Education/educatorinfo.
18. Stith JS, Butterfield WH, Strube MJ, Deusinger SS, Gillespie DF. Personal, interpersonal, and organizational influences on student satisfaction with clinical education. *Phys Ther.* 1998;78:635-645.
19. MacCormick M. The changing role of the nurse teacher. *Nurs Stand.* 1995;10(2):38-41.

3

Type, Amount, and Quality of Clinical Supervision

Thomas G. Weidner, PhD, ATC, FNATA

Why is clinical supervision so important? Because as approved clinical instructor (ACIs)/clinical supervisors, we can positively—or negatively—affect student growth and development. Athletic training students perceive that 53% of their professional development comes from clinical education[1]; hence, we must proactively use our clinical supervision skills. Of course, clinical supervision is a work in progress, both at the local level (ie, in your own clinical settings) and at the national level (ie, interpretation and application of Commission on Accreditation of Athletic Training Education [CAATE] standards). Basically, we now have the opportunity to bring into focus both expected and unexpected outcomes of clinical education reform over the past 10 years. As for expected outcomes, now more than ever our students view themselves as allied health professionals. As for the unexpected, we need to approach clinical supervision with a little more understanding and latitude.

We would do well to view clinical supervision as a triangle with sides consisting of appropriate type, amount, and quality (Figure 3-1).

This chapter aims to help you appreciate current clinical supervision practices regarding these 3 elements. Comments related to best practices regarding clinical supervision will be offered.

TYPE AND AMOUNT OF CLINICAL SUPERVISION

In order to comply with CAATE standards, clinical education must include both clinical experience and clinical education.[2] These two types of instruction are supervised slightly differently.

First, clinical education involves the instruction and approval of clinical proficiencies under the direct supervision of an ACI who has completed appropriate training.[2] Obviously, if an ACI is teaching and evaluating clinical skills and proficiencies, this would require that constant visual and auditory interaction is being maintained between the student and the ACI. This type of clinical education occurs primarily dur-

Figure 3-1. Clinical supervision triangle.

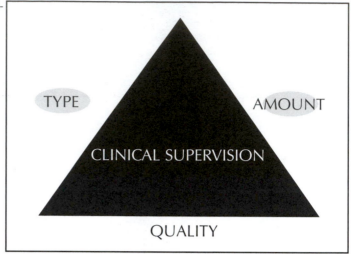

ing the beginning and intermediate phases of the athletic training education program (ATEP). By contrast, primarily advanced students complete clinical experiences under the supervision of a clinical instructor (who may also be an ACI).

These experiences are intended to provide all athletic training students (ATSs) with opportunities to integrate cognitive and psychomotor competencies, clinical proficiencies, and what are now referred to as foundations of professional practice (see Appendix E). These are the core professional behaviors we expect from our students by the completion of the ATEP. During these clinical experiences, the ACI must be physically present, with the ability to intervene on behalf of the patient, while providing ongoing and consistent education for the ATS.[3] Notice that constant visual and auditory interaction as with clinical education is not mentioned here. It is notable, though, that in both types of clinical education, the ACI or clinical instructor is physically present to intervene on behalf of the patient. Now, those students who are unsupervised are not engaged in either type of clinical education and should essentially restrict their activities to those of a first aider.

CURRENT PRACTICES

Perceptions of head athletic trainers and ATSs help to establish a baseline understanding of fairly current supervision practices.[3,4] For these studies, researchers designed a 21-item survey instrument that consists of 3 sections. The first section covers education and athletic program demographics; the second notes first aider qualifications and percentage of time students are supervised during clinical experiences; and the third section examines certified athletic trainer medical coverage and supervision of ATSs during specific moderate risk sports (baseball, field hockey, women's soccer) and increased risk sports (football, wrestling, men's basketball).[5]

More than half of the head athletic trainers indicated that athletic training students provided some medical care coverage without supervision.[3] This included modalities and therapeutic exercise. In contrast, approximately one-third of the students reported that they provided medical care coverage beyond that of a first aider while unsupervised.[4] For both moderate and increased risk sports, head athletic trainers reported that unsupervised students provided a minimal amount of medical care coverage.[3] Perceptions of ATSs varied, however, depending upon the specific moderate or increased risk sport.[4] A rather high percentage (nearly 70%) of head athletic trainers indicated that some of their athletic training students were unsupervised during out-of-town travel with a team.[3] Interestingly, students themselves did not necessarily feel that they were unsupervised as a considerably smaller percentage of students (40%) reported that they traveled with teams without supervision.[4] We assume that these students completed first aider duties only when unsupervised. But of course, as athletes, coaches, and the ATSs themselves all have more expectations than first-aider functions, the responsibilities will likely creep beyond these duties.

At this juncture, it is clear that athletic training students have often been either unsupervised or undersupervised during clinical experiences. One problem with this, beyond CAATE standards and BOC requirements, is that unsupervised or undersupervised athletic training students are not receiving sufficient feedback from a supervisor. ATSs need to know what they are doing right and what they need to work on—both are equally important; the only way to give this feedback is to be there. The right quantity and quality of feedback is paramount to the success of adult learning.[5-7] Nevertheless, one of our obligations as clinical instructors is to encourage independent thinking and problem solving in our students. This is an important step toward professional confidence, and one requiring that we step back from our supervisory roles. Feedback remains crucial, though, even as we strive to engender independence.

The research with head athletic trainers and athletic training students hints at some good trends, too.[3,4] Freshman athletic training students are spending more time in clinical education and direct clinical supervision and less time unsupervised, while senior students are being given more responsibility for decision making. In fact, more advanced students need to be less directly supervised in order to foster their independence, although the ACI must always take into account the health and comfort level of patients and athletes. Athletic training students, at least at some level, are beginning to receive more or less direct clinical supervision depending on their academic standing. Further research should particularly examine to what extent students are being oversupervised during clinical experiences (especially advanced students). Likely, not only are unsupervised or undersupervised clinical experiences markedly diminishing the growth and development of our entry-level professionals, but so too is oversupervision.

It is conceivable that as beginning and intermediate ATSs and ACIs are so often entrenched in direct supervision regarding clinical education, this amount or level of supervision becomes the mode of operation for clinical experience. Use some tough love or tough mentoring with your advanced students and inform them that the expectations are different now. Cast them out further and let them nervously begin making some decisions on their own, interacting with coaches on their own, and the like. See the conclusion of this chapter for more comments regarding the criticality of this matter (Figure 3-2).

Assuming now that the appropriate type and amount of clinical supervision does take place, what do we know about the interactions between ATSs and ACIs that are key to quality clinical supervision? In other words, what is it that we are actually trying to accomplish during clinical supervision? Surely it is more than just preventing or correcting every student mistake. This type of micromanagement would strain ACIs, and have very little lasting impact on our students' professional growth and development.

Researchers identified 4 major categories of helpful and hindering supervisor behaviors.[9] Not surprisingly, students more often reported helpful than hindering behaviors. Mentoring, accepting, nurturing, and modeling behaviors were considered most help-

Figure 3-2. Best practices: Quality of clinical supervision triangle.

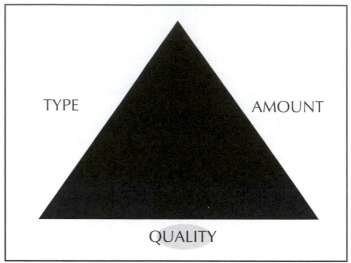

ful. These students reported that they desired to be mentored through explanation, demonstration, and constructive feedback—all quite impossible during unsupervised or undersupervised clinical experiences. They also wanted to be nurtured through confidence building and other supportive supervisor behaviors. Humiliation of the athletic training student and supervisor unavailability (ie, no supervision, undersupervision) were reported to hinder the quality of the clinical experience. Obviously, the quality of the interactions between clinical instructors and students can either positively or negatively affect athletic training student growth and development.

Additional information regarding quality of clinical supervision was revealed in other research.[10] This research identified clinical instructor and athletic training student perceptions of helpful clinical instructor characteristics.

There was high agreement between the students' and clinical instructors' ratings of not only individual items, but also the 10 most helpful and 10 least helpful clinical instructor characteristics. The modeling subgroup contained the most helpful clinical instructor characteristics. Particularly, "displays confidence, manages clinical emergencies well, and demonstrates skills for the students" were perceived by both students and clinical instructors as the most important characteristics. Basically, clinical instructors need to demonstrate and consistently improve their knowledge and skills.

We do know that quality clinical instructors have been described as being both master teachers and master practitioners. Consistent with the modeling behaviors, good clinical instructors have also been identified as being involved with the students, being clear and organized, emphasizing problem solving, mentoring, having sound communication skills, having a positive attitude (sometimes tough under professional role strain), and providing good feedback.

Consider using the Weidner/Henning[10] and the CAATE standards[2] as quality benchmarks. For the former, in a study funded through the NATA Research and Education Foundation (NATAREF), 7 standards and related measurement criteria regarding the ACI's key clinical supervision roles and responsibilities were developed. Three related evaluation forms are available on the NATA Education Council Web site (www.nataec. org).

The 7 Weidner/Henning standards[10] are briefly introduced below (see Chapter 1 for further information).

1. *Legal and ethical behavior*: The ACI needs to hold the appropriate credential (BOC certification; state license, registration, certification, or exemption, if applicable). Perceptions that students form regarding this ethical behavior are important as they face similar requirements in the future. The ACI should also provide athletic training services that are defined by the *Role Delineation Study*[11] and within the scope of the respective state practice act (if applicable).

2. *Communication skills*: The ACI needs to communicate with the program director and/or clinical education coordinator regarding athletic training student progress at regularly scheduled intervals determined by the ATEP.

3. *Interpersonal relationship*: The ACI needs to have an open and approachable demeanor to athletic training students. Relationships which are appropriate and professional should be formed with these students. Again, the ACI should serve as a positive role model and/or mentor in this relationship.

4. *Instructional skills*: The ACI helps athletic training students progress towards meeting the goals and objectives of the clinical experience as assigned by the program director and/or coordinator of clinical education. This is going to include collaborating with these individuals to plan and evaluate learning experiences for students.

5. *Supervisory and administrative skills*: The ACI needs to present clear performance expectations to athletic training students at the beginning and throughout the learning experience. In accordance with CAATE standards,[3] also provide the right type and amount (ie, graded) of clinical supervision.

6. *Evaluation of performance*: The ACI is going to need to note the athletic training student's knowledge, skills, and behaviors as they relate to the goals and objectives of their clinical experience. This will include evaluating student progress during the clinical experience based on performance criteria established by the ATEP. The ACI needs to approach this evaluation process as constructive and educational. Appreciate that ATSs strongly desire feedback.

7. *Clinical skills and knowledge*: The ACI's knowledge and skills need to be current and based on evidence-based medicine (see Chapter 6). The ACI needs to be capable of teaching and evaluating the clinical proficiencies that may be particular to their setting or environment (eg, clinic or corporate setting) as well.

CONCLUSION

For optimal learning, students must be placed in situations that include the appropriate type, amount, and quality of clinical supervision. As your advanced students receive less supervision and feedback (without being placed in positions of ultimate responsibility), their perception of the value of the clinical experience will more likely be that of professional service.[12] This is critical because it is during this time that students are socialized into the profession, acquiring the profession's values and attitudes, interests, skills, and knowledge. Likely at this point they also develop confidence (which tends to be our students' greatest challenge) and develop essential interpersonal and communication skills. Oversupervision of advanced students impedes this progression from student to professional.

Keep in mind the type, amount, and quality of your clinical supervision. Consider strategically using your trusted advanced students to reinforce some clinical education (not clinical experiences) for the beginning students (see Chapter 8). There are enormous benefits for everyone concerned regarding this peer education or peer-assisted learning, including for the busy clinical instructor who has patient care responsibilities.

REFLECTION QUESTIONS

Draw your own insights about your clinical supervision practices by answering these questions:

- Are you appropriately adjusting your supervisory role regarding clinical education and clinical experience with your students?

- Are you under-supervising your students, particularly the beginning and intermediate students?

- Are you over-supervising your students, especially the advanced students?

- Would you consider your supervision practices to be high quality?

REFERENCES

1. Laurent T, Weidner TG. Clinical-education-setting standards are helpful in the professional preparation of employed, entry-level certified athletic trainers. *J Athl Train.* 2002;37(4 Suppl):S248-S254.
2. Commission on Accreditation of Athletic Training Education. *Standards for the accreditation of entry-level athletic training education programs.* Round Rock, TX: Author; 2006.
3. Weidner TG, Pipkin J. Clinical supervision of athletic training students at colleges and universities needs improvement. *J Athl Train.* 2002;37(4 Suppl):S241-S247.
4. Weidner TG, Noble GL, Pipkin JB. Athletic training students in the college/ university setting and the scope of clinical education. *J Athl Train.* 2006;41(4):422-426.
5. Rushton A. Formative assessment: A key to deep learning? *Med Teacher.* 2005;27(6):509-513.
6. Koszalka TA, Ganesan R. Designing online course: a taxonomy to guide strategic use of features available in course Management systems (CMS) in distance edcuation. *Distance Educ.* 2004;25(2):243-256.
7. Charalambos V, Michalinos Z. The design of online learning communities: critical issues. *Education Media International.* 2004;41(2):135-143.
8. Curtis N, Helion JG, Domsohn M. Student athletic trainer perceptions of clinical supervisor behaviors: a critical incident study. *J Athl Train.* 1998;33(3):249-253.
9. Laurent T, Weidner TG. Clinical instructors' and student athletic trainers' perceptions of helpful clinical instructor characteristics. *J Athl Train.* 2001;36(1):58-61.
10. Weidner TG, Henning JM. Importance and applicability of approved clinical instructor standards and criteria to certified athletic trainers in different clinical education settings. *J Athl Train.* 2005;40(4):326-332.
11. Board of Certification. *Role Delineation Study.* 5th ed. Omaha, NE: Author; 2004.
12. Weidner TG, Henning JM. Historical perspective of athletic training clinical education. *J Athl Train.* Dec 2002;37(4 Suppl):S222-S228.

4

Application of Adult Learning Principles in Clinical Teaching

Jolene M. Henning, EdD, ATC, LAT

What are the unique characteristics of adult learners that impact the teaching and learning exchange? Is the typical entry-level athletic training student even considered to be an adult? Do all adults learn the same way or should we utilize a variety of teaching approaches based on the experience of the learner?

These are all questions that most athletic training educators have pondered at one time or another. Fortunately, we have several assumptions about how adults learn that can help provide approved clinical instructors (ACIs) with a framework for clinical teaching. It is important that you begin thinking about such a framework for clinical teaching so that you can better ensure that the strategies you employ will be effective in targeting the needs of the learner. Therefore, this chapter will provide helpful background on constructivist and social learning theories and several assumptions of how adults learn and practical examples of clinical teaching strategies related to these assumptions.

CONSTRUCTIVIST AND SOCIAL LEARNING THEORIES

Athletic training clinical teaching aligns well with the constructivist theory of education in which learning is viewed as an active, student-centered process.[1] The nuts and bolts of constructivism focuses on the student being able to construct meaning from experience, and it is dependent on his or her past knowledge and experiences.[1] In other words, learners should engage in material through hands-on learning and construct their own understanding of clinical concepts by connecting past experiences with new information. As an ACI, your role in the educational process is to facilitate teachable moments in the clinical setting and assist the student with making sense of clinical experiences. This may include helping the student bridge the "theory to practice gap" by applying the concepts that were taught in the classroom and laboratory settings to the clinical setting. For example, your student will gain a deeper understanding of a positive Lachman if he or she can feel it on a patient (rather than just learning about it in the classroom and laboratory).

Social learning theory also has great relevance to clinical education. It accounts for the learner, the environment in which learning takes place, other individuals within that environment, and how all these factors influence one another.[2] Social learning is particularly evident in the clinical setting as the student is "socialized" into the profession. In other words, students learn the norms, values, knowledge, and skills necessary to function as an athletic trainer from their ACIs. So in addition to observing you perform clinical skills, your students are also observing and learning your professional behaviors (eg, communication skills) and personal attributes (eg, honesty, integrity). You provide students with examples of behaviors to copy, modify, or from which to generate new behaviors during their own clinical practices.[3]

ADULT LEARNING

Andragogy, or the art and science of helping adults learn, was introduced by Knowles in the early 1980s.[4,5] Most educational theorists agree that andragogy is less of a theory and more a set of assumptions that guide the practice of teaching adults. In addition, Knowles' ideas of andragogy have received more than their fair share of criticisms. However, we can easily apply its 5 related assumptions (Table 4-1) to improve athletic training clinical teaching.

Self-Directed

The first assumption of andragogy is that adults are independent and self-directed learners. Many of you probably work at institutions whose mission is to develop self-directed, life-long learners. This has become a buzz phrase in higher education, and athletic training is no exception. What does it really mean to be a self-directed learner and how do we encourage our students to develop this trait for life-long learning? Given the educational competencies and clinical proficiencies mandated by accreditation,[6] self-directed learning in its purest sense is not realistic as knowledge and skills are prescribed for the development of an entry-level athletic trainer. However, students can certainly be self-directed within this material. The essence of self-directed learning is that students take ownership in the learning process and can recognize the need, and have the desire, to gain further knowledge and skill. Self-directed learning is certainly a process that can be guided and facilitated by ACIs.

Grow's[7] model of Staged Self-Directed Learning can assist you in guiding your athletic training students (ATSs). The model is based loosely on Hersey and Blanchard's[8] model of situational leadership and includes 4 stages that students progress through when developing self-directedness.

The first stage of self-directed learning is often present in lower-level students who lack knowledge and previous experience but are highly motivated to learn.[7] During this stage, the student is more dependent on the ACI and his or her role is to provide a greater degree of guidance and specific direction. Students in this stage of low self-direction will rely heavily on you as an authority figure. For example, a student engaged in his or her first clinical experience will likely be very enthusiastic about assisting you with duties but will need very specific instructions on how to perform the simplest of tasks (such as restocking a medical kit for practice).

As students learn more about athletic training and gain clinical experience, they progress to the next stage of self-direction. These students are still relatively lack-

TABLE 4-1

FIVE ASSUMPTIONS RELATED TO ADULT LEARNERS

1. As adults mature, they become more self-directed and independent (self-directed).

2. Adults have a reservoir of experience that impacts learning (experience).

3. An adult's readiness to learn is tied to his or her social role (readiness).

4. Adults are problem centered and therefore learning needs to have relevancy and immediate application (problem centered).

5. Adults are motivated more by intrinsic factors than extrinsic factors (motivation).

Adapted from Knowles MS. *The modern practice of adult education: from pedagogy to andragogy.* 2nd ed. New York: Cambridge Books; 1980 and Knowles MS. *The Adult Learner: A Neglected Species.* 3rd ed. Houston, TX: Gulf; 1984.

ing in their foundational knowledge but are becoming more self-motivated to learn more.[7] The ACI can serve as a great motivator and guide for these students by asking clinically relevant questions and encouraging students to look up information on their own. For example, giving your students a question such as, "What is the function of the rotator cuff?" encourages them to seek out information on their own. Similar to stage one, this level of student is also very dependent on the ACI, and is often open to learning everything and anything from you as the keeper of all clinical knowledge!

Students in the third stage of developing self-direction typically have both the basic skill and knowledge to practice clinically but also realize that they need more experience and a deeper understanding of clinical concepts.[7] This is where your role as the ACI becomes critical in fostering self-direction. Consider weekly or biweekly conferences with your students in which you assist them to self-identify learning obstacles and to set specific goals to overcome those obstacles. For example, a student who is lacking confidence in performing an orthopedic evaluation of the hand may be able to self-identify that a lack of understanding regarding the functional anatomy is a key obstacle in performing the evaluation. As the ACI, you can assist the student in setting goals for overcoming this obstacle. This might include a review session with you or a faculty member regarding palpation and biomechanics of the hand, or the student may respond well to simply reviewing course notes on his or her own. The key is to ensure that the student has an opportunity to demonstrate the knowledge/skill resulting from the goal-setting process. This will allow you to provide feedback and ultimately reinforce the need for the student to continue to engage in self-directed learning in the future.

The fourth stage of self-direction occurs when students (often upper-level students) are both willing and able to plan, execute, and evaluate their own learning experiences with or without assistance from an ACI.[7] For example, in developing a rehabilitation plan for a postsurgical type-2 superior labrum from anterior to posterior (SLAP) lesion repair, the student will recognize the need to further understand the implications of this procedure on tissue healing and how the rehabilitation plan needs to differ from that of a type-1 SLAP lesion repair. Ideally, this student will identify the need for additional information (particularly evidence-based medicine) and gather it on his or her own.

Experience

The second assumption of andragogy is that adults have accumulated a wealth of experience that serves as a rich resource for learning. Experience is certainly relative to the level of the student and not all experience leads to learning if it is not coupled with reflection and internalization. In order for learning to occur from previous experiences, the student must be able to connect what he or she has gained from current experiences to past experiences, as well as see implications for what has been learned for future situations. It is very important for you as an ACI to inquire about your student's previous clinical experiences and take advantage of teachable moments that allow for new connections to past experiences. For example, a student who has evaluated a hip injury in a gymnast should be able to recognize the differences in performing this evaluation in a football player, hopefully leading to a new understanding of the nuances in evaluating orthopedic injuries.

Experience, along with developing self-direction, can be viewed within the context of developing supervised student autonomy in the clinical setting. Student autonomy can be viewed along a continuum. There will always be instances in which the student must be dependent on the ACI due to his or her lack of experience and knowledge. Progression along the continuum toward autonomy is highly dependent on the students' clinical skills, their perceived competence in those skills, and their commitment to learning.[9] It would be unwise to assume that because a student has performed independently in a previous situation that he or she would perform with the same level of competence and confidence in a different clinical situation. For example, a student who appears competent and very confident performing an ankle injury evaluation in the athletic training facility may freeze when faced with an acute on-the-field ankle injury. This emphasizes the notion of "spiral learning"[10] or as is described in athletic training as "learning over time."[6] The theory behind spiral learning is that by exposing students to similar clinical experiences (eg, ankle evaluation) in varying clinical contexts (eg, athletic training facility versus on the field), they will be able to discover the important nuances associated with each situation. Or as stated by Bateson,[10] "what was once barely intelligible may be deeply meaningful a second time. And a third." Thus, as students are exposed to more real-time clinical situations, they begin to develop a reservoir of experience from which to enhance their decision-making ability.

In some instances, prior experience can sometimes pose a barrier to learning. For example, in accredited athletic training entry-level master's degree programs it is not uncommon for students to have significant prior clinical experiences (obtained through work-study programs or volunteer experiences at an institution without an accredited program). While these experiences could certainly serve as building blocks for understanding and applying new skills, the contrary can also occur. In other words, students may rely too much on prior experience (observational or hands on) that is often lacking in the corequisite theoretical knowledge that accompanies clinical decision making. For example, a student who has not taken a therapeutic modality course may have observed a certified athletic trainer choose pulsed ultrasound on acute injuries and not understand that it is also used at other times. The ACI (and faculty) will have to further shape the student's understanding of this modality.

Prior experience can also be a barrier to learning if that experience was negative. While we all like to think that we are exceptional ACIs, the reality is that we can unintentionally create a barrier to learning for our students based on our own behaviors. For example, a student may feel that you have insulted him or her in front of a patient. This may be so negative for the student that he or she may become reluctant to interact with patients and apply his or her clinical skills in the future. You may incorrectly interpret this as a lack of knowledge or initiative. Therefore, it is critical that the ACI and student have open communication about expectations and how feedback can be best provided

Readiness

The third assumption of andragogy is that the readiness of adults to learn is closely related to the demands of their "social roles" and daily lives, or in this case the role of being an athletic training student. Students should be tuned into the learning process because their role as an athletic training student depends on learning the required competencies and proficiencies necessary to become certified athletic trainers. A student's readiness to learn is often dependent on his or her emotional maturity, cognitive ability, motivation, experience, confidence, and ability to apply knowledge.[11] Your role is to recognize the student's level of readiness and adapt your teaching strategy accordingly.

Problem Centered

The fourth assumption of andragogy is that adults want to learn information that can be immediately applied in their lives, making them more problem centered than subject centered. This assumption has great implications for clinical teaching and is very much in line with the constructivist theory of learning described previously. Constructivism emphasizes learning through experience and application.[9] Students are more likely to internalize and retain information if they learn it in a manner that focuses on active or hands-on learning. In the clinical setting, this means that students should engage as often as possible in clinical problem solving (at a level that is appropriate for their progression in the academic program). For example, a student may learn more from struggling through his or her first shoulder evaluation than through just observing you perform the evaluation. We all know that the injuries and conditions that may present in the athletic training setting can be very unpredictable. Therefore, it is challenging to teach students everything in "real time" with real patients. It is important to engage students in role playing or patient scenarios to simulate problem solving and clinical application of skills when there is a lack of real-time injuries/conditions in the clinical setting (see Chapter 12 for further comments).

Motivation

The final assumption of andragogy is that adults are more motivated by intrinsic factors than extrinsic influences. It may be that some beginning students appear to lack intrinsic motivation because they are still uncertain about pursuing athletic training as a career. However, one would assume that they would become more intrinsically motivated throughout their development. Knox[12] explains that adults may be intrinsically motivated (and self-directed) because they feel the need to improve their proficiency in a given area in order to improve future job performance. We can relate this to learning isolated skills to performance as a future entry-level athletic trainer. For example, a student may be intrinsically motivated to become more proficient in performing joint mobilizations because a patient in the future may benefit from the technique.

Ideally, students will be intrinsically motivated to learn everything possible during their professional preparation as an athletic trainer. In reality, they may be more motivated by grades, teachers, and their parents' expectations to obtain a degree. You may be able to foster intrinsic motivation through emphasizing the importance of learning clinical skills for enhancing one's decision-making skills. Ideally, students will be able to identify their own areas of weakness and be intrinsically motivated (and self-directed) to improve those clinical skills.

Intrinsic motivation is also a key component in developing lifelong learners. Think about your own motivation to obtain continuing education units (CEUs). Are you extrinsically motivated to develop your knowledge and skills because the BOC requires these CEUs? Or, are you intrinsically motivated to obtain CEUs because you want to improve your clinical performance in certain areas? Likely it is more of the latter. This is something that you can hopefully foster in your students as you model a desire to continue your own education and develop your clinical skills.

REFLECTION QUESTIONS

Draw your own insights about how you can apply educational theory discussed in this chapter into your clinical teaching by answering these questions:

- If an athletic training student appears to be disengaged in the clinical setting, what are some of the possible barriers he or she may be facing? What strategies can you use to help him or her take ownership in the learning process?

- You are supervising a student in his or her final semester of clinical experiences. The student is very dependent on you as the ACI for reassurance and guidance in making clinical decisions. How can you help this student become more self-directed and autonomous?

- Students often appear to lack intrinsic motivation. What teaching strategies can you use to spark motivation?

REFERENCES

1. Bruner J. *Toward a Theory of Instruction.* Cambridge, MA: Harvard University Press; 1966.
2. Bandura AJ. *Social Learning Theory.* New York: General Learning Press; 1971.
3. Bahn D. Social learning theory: Its application in the context of nurse education. *Nurse Educ Today.* 2001;21:110-117.
4. Knowles MS. *The Modern Practice of Adult Education: From Pedagogy to Andragogy.* 2nd ed. New York: Cambridge Books; 1980.
5. Knowles MS. *The Adult Learner: A Neglected Species.* 3rd ed. Houston: Gulf; 1984.
6. Commission on Accreditation of Athletic Training Education. Standards for the Accreditation of Entry-level Athletic Training Education Programs. Retrieved November 7, 2008m from: http://caate.net/documents/standards.6.30.08.pdf.
7. Grow G. Teaching learners to be self-directed: a stage approach. *Adult Education Quarterly.* 1991; 41(3):125-129.
8. Hersey P, Blanchard K. *Management and Organizational Behavior: Utilizing Human Resources.* 5th ed. Englewood Cliffs, NJ: Prentice Hall; 1988.
9. Merriam SB, Caffarella RS. *Learning in Adulthood.* 2nd ed. San Francisco, CA: Jossey-Bass; 1999.
10. Bateson MC. *Peripheral Visions: Learning Along the Way.* New York: Harper Collins; 1994.
11. Meyer LP. Athletic training clinical instructors as situational leaders. *J Athl Train.* 2002;37(4 Suppl): S261-S265.
12. Knox AB. Proficiency theory of adult learning. *Contemporary Educational Psychology.* 1980;5:378-404.

5

Teaching and Learning Styles During Clinical Education

Jolene M. Henning, EdD, ATC, LAT

Suppose a new therapeutic modality unit came out tomorrow with all the latest bells and whistles. How would you go about learning it?

- Would you read the instructor's manual cover to cover to learn about each unique feature?
- Would you use the quick start menu on the touch screen and learn the rest as you go?
- Would you invite an expert to provide you with an in-service?
- Would you call a colleague who has the new unit and ask him or her how to use it?
- Would you base your understanding of the unit on the older model?

The point is that all of these strategies will eventually lead to learning how to use the unit. There is not one right or better approach when the end result is the same, but you may have a preference for one approach over another. This preference is often referred to as a learning style. Just like you have preferred ways of learning new information through continuing education, your students have preferred ways of learning in the clinical setting. The purpose of this chapter is to define learning styles, examine the learning characteristics and challenges identified by 3 commonly used learning style inventories, and illustrate the application of specific teaching strategies that address different learning styles during clinical education.

WHAT ARE LEARNING STYLES?

Have you ever wondered why it is easier to teach some students more than others? Have you ever told a student to go home and look up information about a rehabilitation protocol and be prepared for questions the next day only to be frustrated that the student did not grasp the information? Part of the challenge may be related to a difference in learning styles. While as a lifelong learner you may have developed an inclination for looking up information as needed, a young athletic training student (ATS) may have a stronger preference for learning about such information directly from an expert—you!

Learning styles are preferred modes that are used to learn, produce, solve problems, and achieve results. No person has a single learning style but rather fluidly moves in and out of preferred modes of learning depending on different situations. It can be helpful to have your students complete a learning style inventory at the beginning of their clinical rotation in order to gain insight into their preferred modes of learning. Caution should be used, however, to avoid pigeon holing a student into one method of learning. Athletic training education research clearly indicates that there is not one dominant learning style among ATSs.[1] There is also little relationship between a student's learning style and his or her success on the BOC examination.[2]

It is important to understand how your students learn best in order to have the most effective teaching and learning exchange. To better illustrate this point, let us consider the athletic training student as part of your athletic health care team. As the team leader, you need to not only be aware of the styles of your team members but of your own preferred style as well. For example, if you consistently run into a dead end with a student when trying to emphasize the sense of urgency that exists in certain clinical situations, it may be necessary to alter your approach with that student. It is critical to have a cadre of strategies that you could implement to address your students' fluid learning styles.

LEARNING STYLE INVENTORIES

There are many learning style inventories that have been developed over the years that help to explain students' preferred modes to acquire information. I will discuss two commonly used inventories in athletic training education, as well as take a brief look at the research in our field related to these instruments.

Kolb Learning Style Inventory

Dr. David Kolb[3] began developing the Kolb Learning Style Inventory (LSI) in the early 1970s in an attempt to explain how people learn best. His LSI is based on a cycle of learning that involves a concrete experience or event, reflective observation, abstract conceptualization or thinking, and active experimentation or decision making and problem solving. The cycle starts again with another concrete experience that results from the decisions made in the previous cycle.[3] This model of using experience as the impetus for learning led to the categorization of preferred modes of learning based on these cycles. Table 5-1 explores the characteristics and challenges of the 4 types of learners as described by Kolb: converger, diverger, assimilator, and the accommodator.[4,5]

Converger

Convergers approach learning in a logical manner, taking a systematic approach that is focused on problem solving.[6] These learners tend to be self-directed but not particularly collaborative in the learning process.[6] On the positive side, they will not be afraid to jump in and make clinical decisions and attempt to solve problems. It may be productive to work with this student who takes initiative to complete technical tasks. The challenge, however, is that the student may have tunnel vision and focus on solving a problem without taking all of the pertinent details into account. For example, when conducting a shoulder assessment, the student may be so focused on reaching a clinical diagnosis of impingement syndrome that he or she fails to consider all of

TABLE 5-1

CHARACTERISTICS FROM KOLB'S LEARNING STYLE INVENTORY

LEARNING STYLE	CHARACTERISTICS	CHALLENGES
Converger	*Decision maker* Takes abstract information and processes concrete solutions	May prematurely make a decision or rush to solve a problem without all necessary information
Diverger	*Creator* Takes in information from concrete experience and processes *Brainstorming* Imagination allows for creation of many alternative solutions	Can become overwhelmed by alternatives and indecisiveness through observation May have difficulty prioritizing tasks
Assimilator	*Systematic planner* *Goal setter* Takes in abstract information and observations to create a rational explanation *Inductive reasoner*	Tends to create "castles in the air" May be impractical May prematurely discuss solutions without all critical facts
Accommodator	*Do-er* Learns through practical experience Adapts to change Transforms concrete information into action	May be pushy or impatient Too much time on trivial tasks

Adapted from: N/A. One style doesn't fit all. The different ways people learn and why it matters. Retrieved July 2, 2008, from: http://www.haygroup.com/tl/Downloads/Why_People_Learn.pdf and Kolb AY, Kolb DA. The Kolb Learning Style Inventory Version 3.1: 2005 Technical Specifications. Case Western Reserve University. May 15, 2005.

the contributing factors that have led to the development of the symptoms. His or her focus is on "Look, I have an answer" rather than identifying all of the factors that would need to be addressed in treating and rehabilitating this patient. He or she could easily fall into the trap of treating symptoms rather than causes. In a situation like this, your role as the ACI is to ensure that the student has gathered all of the details and can articulate reasons for his or her decision based on objective clinical data.

Diverger

Divergers often prefer to observe others performing clinical skills before attempting them on their own.[6] As the ACI, you will spend more time modeling or demonstrating skills to divergers before they are comfortable attempting tasks on their own. Divergers tend to be very thorough clinicians and want to view clinical problems through multiple perspectives to ensure that no stone goes unturned. They can be a great resource for brainstorming solutions to clinical problems that are not obvious or are atypical. The challenge with this type of student, however, is that thoroughness can sometimes interfere with the sense of urgency that exists in many situations. For example, I have observed students that get so focused on conducting a thorough on-the-field evaluation, that they get side-tracked by irrelevant information and lose focus on what the patient is sharing. You may have had students in the athletic training room attempt to conduct their first injury evaluation and find that they are performing every special test in the book, regardless of relevancy to the current situation. This can be characteristic of a diverger. However, also keep in mind that this is also a normal developmental process that students (regardless of learning style) go through in becoming a more efficient clinician. It will take a while before they can determine what information is pertinent and what does not apply. Your role as the ACI is to be patient and offer specific feedback to the student as to why certain tasks are not relevant to his or her particular situation. For example, it would be important to have your student articulate his or her rationale for why he or she performed a complete lower quarter screening on a patient who clearly had the mechanism for an anterior cruciate ligament (ACL) tear. This simple act of reflection and articulation can often be very eye opening for your students as you help them to see the big picture.

Another potential challenge with divergers is their difficulty with multi-tasking, which we would all agree is a critical skill as an athletic trainer. This difficulty often lies in their desire to be thorough and their tendency to become overwhelmed by alternatives thus, impacting their ability to prioritize. Imagine how a diverger must feel the first time there are 3 patients who need care at one time. Your role is to help him or her prioritize this care. For example, let's say these 3 patients arrive for rehabilitation at the same time. Help the student to realize that the patient who needs to warm up on the bike should begin that activity; meanwhile, you set up another patient on electrical stimulation, and thus leave time for the third patient who needs more hands-on care. We could explore countless examples of multi-tasking in the athletic training setting that would be overwhelming for a diverger. This type of prioritization has probably become natural for you as a seasoned clinician, but to a novice student it is a skill that must be developed. The key is for you to recognize when students are frustrated and guide them through developing priorities.

Assimilator

Assimilators are often very proficient in understanding a theoretical or evidence-based approach to clinical practice. However, they can easily get lost in theory and attempt to "reinvent the wheel." They also may lack the ability to transfer theory into practical application. These students often prefer to work alone and view the ACI as the expert. Therefore, group activities and peer-assisted learning may not be the most effective strategies for reaching these students. A more effective approach would be the use of individual case studies that allow the student to delve into a problem for thorough independent exploration. Assimilators will enjoy reading research and exploring additional information that relates to injuries/conditions they have encountered in the clinical setting.

Accommodator

Accommodators are often very practical and action-oriented students. They are risk takers who jump into clinical situations to get their hands dirty and ask questions later. They are often the first students to volunteer for about any task just so they have something to do. The down side is that they can become so overly focused on completing these trivial tasks that they miss out on more valuable learning opportunities.

Accommodators work well with others and learn best through practical experience. However, they can become frustrated during "down time" when there is little action. In such instances, consider using peer-assisted learning (see Chapter 8 for more information), role playing, and clinical simulations.[6] These are very effective strategies for teaching these students because they allow them to continue to engage in active learning when nothing may be happening in real time.

Accommodators need to be constantly challenged with new experiences. As an ACI, this can be both a blessing and a curse. This type of student will be a sponge in the clinical setting and will want to learn *how* to do everything you are doing but not necessarily *why* you are doing it. Caution should be used with this type of student when teaching new clinical skills because he or she will have a tendency to prematurely rush into the application of a new skill on a patient without the appropriate level of practice or foundational knowledge for its application.

Another potential challenge with this type of learner is his or her tendency to become pushy or impatient for action. As a result, the student may not completely think through his or her decisions. On the positive side, however, accommodators often have great clinical instincts that can often be difficult to foster in students. Therefore, asking the student for the "gut feelings" can be an effective approach in validating his or her thought processes.[6]

Athletic Training Education Research Regarding Kolb Learning Style Inventory

While research in athletic training using the Kolb Learning Style Inventory (LSI) has not identified one dominate learning style, there appears to be trends in how students prefer to learn. In one study, approximately 30% of athletic training students were accommodators and 30% were assimilators.[7] In another study, approximately 38% of athletic training students were classified as assimilators with relatively equal distribution of students falling into the other 3 categories.[1] Another study examined learning style differences in the classroom versus clinical settings and found that students have different preferred modes of learning in each setting.[8] Coker[8] found that the predominant learning styles in the clinical setting were converger and accommodator (42.3% and 30.8%, respectively). However, in the classroom setting, the predominant learning styles were assimilator (65.4%) and converger (15.4%). What this all means for the ACI is that you need a "bag of tricks" to address a wide variety of learning styles in your students.

Gregorc Style Delineator

Dr. Anthony Gregorc[9] uses a different approach to examine learning preferences that is based on his theory of mind styles. Gregorc's theory is centered around the constructs or concepts of perception and ordering, in other words, how information is grasped and then arranged, referenced, and disposed.[9] The construct of perception is categorized along a continuum ranging from abstract to concrete.[10] Abstractness refers to perceiving information through reason, emotion, and intuition.[10] Concreteness refers to individuals whose perceptions rely on visual, auditory, and tactile senses.[10] The construct or concept of ordering is arranged along a continuum from sequence to randomness and relates to how new information is processed.[10] Individuals functioning on the sequential end of the continuum utilize linear, methodical, and systematic methods for ordering new information. For example, these individuals prefer step-by-step directions for completing tasks. Individuals functioning on the random end of the continuum employ a more holistic, unstructured, and nonlinear approach to ordering new information and do not rely on a sequential approach to learning.[9,10] The associated Gregorc Style Delineator measures the processing and ordering constructs described above, resulting in 4 different combinations of mind styles: concrete sequential, abstract sequential, concrete random, and abstract random. Similar to the

Kolb LSI, one can assume that students have abilities in each of these styles but may lean more toward one style than the others as they complete their clinical experiences. The characteristics and challenges of working with students with these different mind styles are presented in Table 5-2.[11]

Concrete Sequential

Concrete sequential learners prefer structured learning environments that lean towards being predictable. You should work with the student to create a weekly schedule that clearly indicates your expectations of when he or she should be in the athletic training clinic. Students of this nature will likely not respond well to unexpected changes in practice schedules, although this usually cannot be avoided. It is also a good idea to spell out your expectations for the student in writing at the beginning of his or her clinical experience. This will avoid any confusion about policies and procedures in the future.

Concrete sequential learners also prefer hands-on experience and will often take an orderly approach to completing tasks. They often strive for perfection. You may find that more novice students are dominant concrete sequential learners because they are lacking in foundational knowledge. They take a very systematic approach to learning and their perspective is, "Tell me *exactly* how to do it and I will perfect it." When teaching new skills to these students, it is helpful to provide them with a step-by-step approach from beginning to end, a process known as forward lengthening. For example, when teaching a student how to perform gait analysis, it is helpful to have a written list of all the steps you intend to evaluate. Model each one systematically, and allow the student to practice each step. Another approach for this type of learner is a process called backward chaining in which you begin teaching a skill by demonstrating the complete process and then breaking the skill down into its sequential parts. For example, when teaching a student how to construct custom orthotics, it is helpful to begin with a completed product so they can visualize what the end result should look like. This will help students visualize the steps necessary to reach the outcome.

Concrete sequential learners often seek out answers that are black and white and can become frustrated when there is more than one answer or multiple ways to complete a task. You may hear this type of student say "that is not the way we learned it in lab" or "My previous ACI did not do it that way." It can be particularly challenging for these students when there is not an obvious answer to a clinical problem. They will become frustrated in attempting to reach a clinical diagnosis for an injury that is not clear cut. Developing differential diagnoses can be good practice for these students. Another example is that these students can become overwhelmed understanding rehabilitation progression. They may view a rehabilitation protocol as too vague because it focuses on patient guidelines and goals rather than specific exercises, sets, and reps. For example, engage them in brainstorming to identify all possible exercises that fit the guideline of "initiate scapular stabilizer strengthening" in phase 2 rehabilitation of a Bankart repair.

Abstract Sequential

Abstract sequential learners are highly analytical and can extrapolate meaning from observations. They mentally outline the necessary steps to complete a task without specific written instructions. Teaching strategies that work well with these students include verbal instructions while modeling skills. They would rather observe the expert ACI perform a task before attempting the skill themselves. Abstract sequential learners prefer using visual aids (eg, anatomical models) as well as to complete independent reading.

TABLE 5-2

CHARACTERISTICS FROM GREGORC'S MIND STYLES INVENTORY

MIND STYLE	CHARACTERISTICS	CHALLENGES
Concrete sequential	Work systematically Expectations need to be clear Very organized Established routine Literal interpretations Apply ideas in practical way	Unorganized environment Unclear directions Questions with no right or wrong answer Working in groups Working with unpredictable people
Abstract sequential	Gathers information before making a decision Learns by watching more than doing Wants to learn from the expert Uses exact well-researched information Figures out what needs to be done Very thorough	Working with those with a different view Too little time to deal with situation thoroughly Difficulty expressing emotion Repetitive tasks become boring Often monopolizes a conversation
Concrete random	Sees many options and solutions Risk taker Thinks fast on his or her feet Inspires others to take action Accepts many types of people and viewpoints Learns from real world experience Works under general time frames	Restrictions and limitations Routines Keeping detailed records Formal reports Having no options Having to choose only one option Explaining how he or she made a decision
Abstract random	Listens well to others Understands feelings and emotions Brings harmony to group situations Establishes positive relationships Enthusiastic participation in projects he or she believes in Likes personalized learning Decisions made with heart instead of head	Having to justify feelings Does not like competition Working with dictatorial personalities Working in a restrictive environment Working with unfriendly people Multitasking Accepting criticism

Adapted from Mills DW. Applying what we know student learning styles. http://www.csrnet.org/csrnet/articles/student-learning-styles.html. Accessed July 2, 2008.

As these students are very thorough and analytical, they easily become frustrated when there is not sufficient time. Your role is to assist these students in improving their efficiency in the clinical setting. One tactic is to actually time the student in how long it takes to perform a clinical task (such as an injury scenario) and then have the student reflect and analyze on which components proved to be unnecessary. This type of time-restricted activity may prove to be frustrating but necessary in order to improve their clinical efficiency without sacrificing thoroughness. Abstract sequential learners also enjoy learning through discussion. However, they tend to dominate the conversation and become frustrated when others have differing opinions. As a result, discussions with their ACIs are much more productive than those with their peers.

Concrete Random

Concrete random learners are intuitive and insightful risk takers that will often be viewed as leaders by their peers. These students quickly catch on to clinical problem-solving and often skip steps in making decisions. The key is not to chastise the student for skipping steps, but rather ask for his or her rationale on why certain steps were skipped. You might find that they are operating at a higher level of critical thinking and skipping over certain steps was completely justified. These students will excel in leadership positions and peer leadership opportunities should be fostered to enhance their learning (see Chapter 7 for more information).

Students who are concrete random dominant prefer to learn by trial and error and do not like to have their options limited. This can create a tricky situation for you as their ACI. The students' trial and error approach certainly signifies initiative and motivation that you do not want to hamper. However, you have an obligation to your patients to ensure that no harm is done by the student. The best approach is to allow the student to "experiment" with his or her patient care and intervene if his or her choices will cause harm. Reserve your feedback until the student has completed the task. This will give your student an opportunity for further exploration and reflection. More than likely, the student will already be acutely aware of what worked and what did not.

These students thrive in a busy environment. However, you may need to remind them about routine tasks. They do not enjoy mundane or repetitive tasks such as restocking medical kits or updating patient records. In order to emphasize the importance of completing such tasks, it is helpful to utilize simulations or role playing that illustrates what can happen if they are not completed. For example, a mock emergency scenario will certainly point out the potential deleterious effects of not having enough supplies in your medical kit to control bleeding. To underline the importance of record keeping, you could create a scenario that involves a rejected insurance claim because the student failed to keep adequate records. The more you can actively engage these learners in situations that stress the "real world" of athletic training, the more likely they will internalize the information and appreciate its importance.

Abstract Random

Abstract random learners work well with others and are good listeners. They are not competitive in nature and function best in non-hostile environments that are easy-going. They do not respond well to ACIs with strong, dictatorial personalities. These students will tend to focus on establishing positive relationships with their patients and value a holistic approach to patient care. They may have a tendency to become overly involved with, or attached to, their patients. The need for maintaining professional boundaries will need to be emphasized.

Abstract random learners often have difficulty accepting criticism. Therefore, it is essential to provide constructive feedback that is specific to their actions rather than vague and which could be interpreted as a personal attack on their character. These learners also need time to process new information and reflect on their performance. Therefore, providing feedback too early can be detrimental. It is better to allow the student to complete a task rather than interrupting. Provide feedback away from the patient.

Athletic Training Education Research Regarding the Gregorc Style Delineator

Compared to the Kolb LSI, little athletic training education research has been conducted regarding the Gregorc Style Delineator. Gould and Caswell[12] compared mind styles of undergraduate athletic training students with that of program directors. The concrete sequential mind style was the predominant style (63.4%) in both students and program directors, regardless of sex or the student's year in the program. Abstract random was the second most dominant style (approximately 40%), with female students having a higher preference for this style than males. There is some research that suggests that students who choose science-based fields are more likely to have concrete sequential mind styles[10] and therefore it is not surprising that athletic training students seem to follow this same trend.

CONCLUSION

Learning styles can be useful in identifying how students may react in a particular learning situation. They are fluid and can vary as a student progresses throughout their clinical education. It will be helpful to you as the ACI to be aware of how you prefer to learn and how your own learning preference may interact with your students' preferences. Being aware of potential incongruence in styles may help you more effectively adapt your clinical teaching for different students.

REFLECTION QUESTIONS

Draw your own insights about whether you are adapting your clinical teaching based on your students' learning styles by answering these questions:

- Identify 3 ways to effectively teach students in the clinical setting who are categorized as assimilators. How would you change your approach if you were also supervising an accommodator?

- You are supervising a concrete sequential sophomore athletic training student who is very intimidated about applying basic clinical skills on real patients. When questioning the student about how to perform such skills, she appears to have a grasp on the foundational knowledge. How can you assist this student in making the transition from knowledge to application?

REFERENCES

1. Brower KA, Stemmans CL, Ingersoll CD, Langley DJ. An investigation of undergraduate athletic training students' learning styles and program admission success. *J Athl Train.* 2001;36(2):130–135

2. Draper DO. Students' learning styles compared with their performance on the NATA certification exam. *Athl Train.* 1989;24:234–235,275.

3. Kolb DA. *Experiential Learning: Experience as the Source of Learning and Development.* Englewood Cliffsl, NJ: Prentice Hall; 1984.

4. One style doesn't fit all. The different ways people learn and why it matters. http://www.haygroup.com/tl/Downloads/Why_People_Learn.pdf. Accessed July 2, 2008.

5. Kolb AY, Kolb DA. The Kolb Learning Style Inventory Version 3.1: 2005 Technical Specifications. Case Western Reserve University. May 15, 2005

6. Beresford J. Teaching strategies for effective learning. In *Matching Teaching to Learning*. London: Optimus Education; 5–16.

7. Stradley SL, Buckley BD, Kaminski TW, Horodyski MB, Fleming D, Janelle CM. A nationwide learning-style assessment of undergraduate athletic training students in CAAHEP-accredited athletic training programs. *J Athl Train.* 2002;37(4 Supplement):S-141–S-146.

8. Coker CA. Consistency of learning styles of undergraduate athletic training students in the traditional classroom versus the clinical setting. *J Athl Train.* 2000;35:441–444.

9. Gregorc AF. *An Adult's Guide to Style.* Maynard, MA: Gabriel Systems Inc; 1982.

10. Seidel LE, England EM. Gregorc's cognitive styles: college students' preferences for teaching methods and testing techniques. *Perceptual and Motor Skills.* 1999;88:859–875.

11. Mills DW. *Applying what we know student learning styles.* http://www.csrnet.org/csrnet/articles/student-learning-styles.html. Accessed July 2, 2008.

12. Gould TE, Caswell SV. Stylistic learning differences between undergraduate athletic training students and educators: Gregorc mind styles. *J Athl Train.* 2006;41:109–116.

6

Incorporating and Teaching Evidence-Based Practice

Lisa S. Jutte, PhD, ATC, LAT and Stacy E. Walker, PhD, ATC, LAT

You have the opportunity to impact many patients' and students' lives, as an athletic trainer and as an approved clinical instructor (ACI). During their clinical experiences, students model and learn through the behaviors of their ACIs. One skill you can model for students, and improve your patient care, is applying evidence-based medicine (EBM) to your clinical practice. EBM is a relatively new term. It was coined in 1992 by physicians from McMaster University.[1] You may see the terms *EBM* and *evidence-based practice* (EBP) often used interchangeably, but they are different. EBP is the specific way you make decisions regarding the evaluation, diagnosis, and treatment of your patient, while EBM is using the evidence to support such practice. Since 1992, there has been an explosion of training programs (eg, courses, workshops, seminars) to educate health professionals about this new paradigm.[2] Today, a search for EBM and EBP in PubMed reveals more than 70,000 citations.

The objective of EBP is to incorporate the most current and valid medical information available into your clinical practice. Using current evidence can help you improve your patient diagnoses and treatments.[3] This can help ensure that you are providing quality care and reducing the number of unsuccessful and unwarranted treatments (while saving time and resources). EBP should not replace your clinical expertise or be overly time consuming. Unfortunately, some training programs leave the impression that EBM requires hours of study to answer a single patient care question.[4] Reading the wrong material faster or spending a significant amount of time reading does not mean one is acquiring more knowledge.[5] In this chapter, we will discuss the concepts of EBM and EBP; the steps required to practice EBM; and how to introduce, demonstrate, and assess the skills your students need to practice EBP.

UNDERSTANDING EVIDENCE-BASED MEDICINE AND EVIDENCE-BASED PRACTICE

You need EBM to make EBP possible. EBM is described as "the integration of the best research evidence with our clinical expertise and with our patient's unique values and circumstances."[2] Best research refers to valid and clinically relevant research relating to the patient's circumstance. For example, if a 15-year-old high school baseball pitcher presents with a possible rotator cuff tear, you could search the medical literature to determine the best method for diagnosis.[6] Clinical expertise refers to your past experience in evaluating, treating, and rehabilitating injuries and illnesses and integrating that experience into your current decisions regarding patient care. In our example, a novice athletic trainer may not have any prior experience treating a 15-year-old with a rotator cuff injury, but a seasoned clinician may have treated many patients with rotator cuff injuries in this age group. An athletic trainer's past experiences should logically influence how he or she manages his or her current patients. Lastly, patients' values and circumstances refer to the unique expectations and situation of each patient. For example, a high school senior athlete who plans to play sports in college could have different values and expectations regarding his or her care than another senior who will not continue to play competitively in college sports. In addition, the athlete's parents may have different treatment expectations based on health insurance restrictions or their own desire for their child to receive a college athletic scholarship. All of these factors that constitute best research, clinical expertise, and patients' values and circumstances are equally important and must be taken into account when evaluating, diagnosing, and treating your patients. The total integration of EBM into clinical practice is referred to as EBP.

APPROVED CLINICAL INSTRUCTORS ARE CRUCIAL IN TEACHING AND MODELING EVIDENCE-BASED PRACTICE

As an ACI, you not only assist students in learning EBM but you also inspire students to use EBP. If students are only exposed to EBP during their didactic instruction, they are less likely to integrate EBP into their future clinical practice.[7] Teaching EBP in the clinical setting, as compared to just in the classroom, has a greater impact on a student's future ability and willingness to practice EBP.[8] Students are more likely to change their skill, attitude, and behavior toward EBP based on their clinical experiences.[8] Therefore, as an ACI, you play a critical role in a student's education regarding EBP.

TEACHING THE CONCEPT OF EVIDENCE-BASED PRACTICE

Before students can begin EBP, they must understand what it is and the role it plays in clinical practice. It may or may not become your responsibility to provide your athletic training students (ATSs) with the initial introduction to EBP, but regardless they must first understand the concept. If your students are unfamiliar with the concept of EBP, here are 3 strategies you can use to teach them about EBP:

TABLE 6-1

EVIDENCE-BASED MEDICINE INTRODUCTORY TOOLS, ARTICLES, ONLINE TUTORIALS, AND WEB SITES

Bigby M. Evidence-based medicine in a nutshell: a guide to finding and using the best evidence in caring for patients. *Arch Dermatol.* 1998;134:1609-1618.

Ciliska D. Educating for evidence-based practice. *J Prof Nurs.* 2005;21:345-350.

Haynes BR. Of studies, summaries, synopses, and systems: the "4S" evolution of services for finding current best evidence. *Evid Based Ment Health.* 2001;4:37-38.

Khan KS, Coomarasamy A. A hierarchy of effective teaching and learning to acquire competence in evidenced-based medicine. *BMC Med Ed.* 2006;6:59.

1. Discuss EBP and provide examples as to how your clinical practice has changed based on evidence. Some examples may include updates in cardiopulmonary resuscitation CPR, use of automated external defibrillators (AEDs), concussion diagnosis, and/or treatment of heat illness.

2. Assign your students to read an article on EPB or EBM and then discuss it with them. You could use any one of several articles listed in Table 6-1.

3. Ask your students to complete a web-based tutorial on EBP or EBM (Table 6-2). Many university libraries and/or medical schools provide free Web-based tutorials. These tutorials are usually developed for physicians, but the concepts and practice are similar for any health care professional.

Any or all of the above strategies can help you introduce the concept of EBP and also facilitate some very interesting dialogue with your students.

FIVE STEPS OF EVIDENCE-BASED PRACTICE

Once your students have an understanding of EBM, they can begin to learn the 5 steps of EBP, which include the following[2]:

1. Asking a clinical question based on the need for information

2. Researching the best evidence which relates to the clinical question

3. Critically evaluating the validity, impact, and applicability of the evidence

4. Applying the evidence to the clinical problem in the context of your clinical expertise and the patient's values and circumstances

5. Evaluating the effectiveness of the previous steps, and seeking ways to improve evaluation, treatment, etc of your patients for the future

As we describe each of these steps in the remainder of this chapter, please keep in mind that experts suggest teaching the steps in sequential small doses due to the complexity of EBP.[9]

TABLE 6-2

LIST OF EVIDENCE-BASED MEDICINE TUTORIALS

Tutorial Name	Host Institution	Web Address
Introduction to Evidence-Based Medicine, 4th edition	Duke University Medical Center Library and Health Sciences Library, UNC-Chapel Hill	www.hsl.unc.edu/services/tutorials/ebm/welcome.htm
Introduction to Evidence-Based Medicine	Alumni Medical Library Boston University Medical Center	http://medlib.bu.edu/tutorials/ebm/intro/index.cfm?loc=ebmwiki
Introduction to Information Mastery	Michigan State University Department of Family Practice	www.poems.msu.edu/InfoMastery/
Searching the Literature for Medical Evidence*	University of California San Francisco School of Medicine	http://missinglink.ucsf.edu/lm/EBM_litsearch/index.html
Understanding Evidence-Based Healthcare: A Foundation for Action	United States Cochrane Center	http://apps1.jhsph.edu/cochrane/CUEwebcourse.htm
PubMed Tutorial*	National Library of Medicine	www.nlm.nih.gov/bsd/pubmed_tutorial/m1001.html
A Student's Guide to the Medical Literature*	University of Colorado Health Sciences Center	http://grinch.uchsc.edu/sg/index.html
Evidence-Based Clinical Practice Tutorial	University of Rochester Medical Center	www.urmc.rochester.edu/hslt/miner/resources/evidence_based/
Practicing EBM	Centre for Evidence-Based Medicine, University Health Network & University of Toronto Libraries	www.cebm.utoronto.ca/parctise

*Also includes tutorials on literature searches

Step 1: Teaching Students to Ask Clinical Questions

Asking well-constructed clinical questions is the cornerstone of EBP. ATSs need to understand how to develop clinical questions before they can efficiently find relevant medical evidence. As an ACI, you may already encourage students to ask questions. Developing a clinical question is not much different from the questions your ATSs may

TABLE 6-3

PICO—A METHOD FOR CONSTRUCTING CLINICAL QUESTIONS

		TYPE OF INFORMATION INCLUDED FOR EACH CRITERIA	PICO COMPONENTS FOR A DIAGNOSTIC* QUESTION BASED ON ROTATOR CUFF PATIENT EXAMPLE	PICO COMPONENTS FOR A TREATMENT† QUESTION BASED ON ROTATOR CUFF PATIENT EXAMPLE
P	Patient or Problem	Age Gender Race Information about disease or primary complaint	15-year-old male baseball pitcher complaining of shoulder pain	15-year-old male baseball pitcher complaining of shoulder pain
I	Intervention	Diagnostic tests Refer patient Treatment	Diagnostic ultrasound	Surgical repair
C	Comparison	Alternative intervention	Magnetic resonance angiography	Therapeutic rehabilitation or no treatment
O	Outcome	Pain relief Decrease swelling Increased range of motion Increased strength Increased function	Correct diagnosis	Functional return to play

*Diagnostic Clinical Question: Does diagnostic ultrasound provide a more accurate diagnosis than MRI for rotator cuff injuries in adolescent athletes?

†Treatment Clinical Question: In an adolescent athlete with a rotator cuff tear, will surgical repair result in better function than rehabilitation alone?

already be asking during their clinical experiences. The PICO method can be used for developing these questions, and contains 4 criteria (Patient or Problem, Intervention, Comparison, and Outcome).[10,11] The patient or problem criteria describes a specific characteristic of the patient and/or problem. The intervention is the treatment or evaluation techniques about which you want to learn more. The comparison is another treatment or evaluation technique for which you would like to compare the intervention, and it may be no treatment. Lastly, the outcome is how the intervention will be assessed. The PICO method is useful for helping your student to develop and focus a complete clinical question. This will include specifying information regarding the patient, treatment options, and outcomes of interest. Clinical questions need to be specific in order to narrow your search for evidence. An example of the PICO method for 2 clinical questions can be found in Table 6-3.

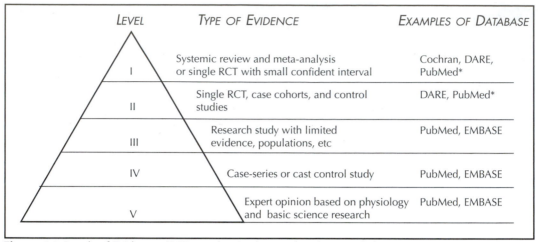

LEVEL	TYPE OF EVIDENCE	EXAMPLES OF DATABASE
I	Systemic review and meta-analysis or single RCT with small confident interval	Cochran, DARE, PubMed*
II	Single RCT, case cohorts, and control studies	DARE, PubMed*
III	Research study with limited evidence, populations, etc	PubMed, EMBASE
IV	Case-series or cast control study	PubMed, EMBASE
V	Expert opinion based on physiology and basic science research	PubMed, EMBASE

Figure 6-1. Levels of Evidence. (RCT=randomized control trial, * search for systematic reviews or meta-analysis.)

To help teach students how to ask clinical questions, consider using the following strategies:

- Ask students to develop a clinical question from a current case on which you are working. You can review the question using the PICO method and discuss whether the question satisfies each criterion.

- Use a common patient problem from your setting that you would like to investigate (should another patient present with a similar injury/condition in the future) (eg, a wrester with a skin condition or a football player with a concussion).

- Examine a previous case and assess if current information would change how you would manage that patient today.

Encourage your students to use the PICO method to develop clinical questions whenever possible. With practice, developing well-structured clinical questions will become second nature.

Step 2: Teaching Students to Research Medical Evidence

Once your students are able to formulate clinical questions, your next step is to research appropriate medical evidence to help answer those questions. They will need to understand the hierarchy or levels of evidence. This includes knowing that specific levels of information are found from specific sources and that the level of evidence indicates how much credence you should give to the results.

Levels of Medical Evidence

The level of medical evidence refers to the categorization of evidence ranked according to the strength and validity of that evidence. The levels help indicate how useful it will be to answer your clinical question. Medical evidence ranges from the lowest level, expert opinion and basic science research (level V), to case reports, case series (level IV), to clinical research (level III), to clinical research with outcome measures and randomized control trials (RCT) with larger confidence intervals (level II) to meta-analyses and systematic reviews (level I) (Figure 6-1). Level I evidence is considered superior because it incorporates the results from several randomized control trials using real patients, thereby reducing bias and testing the research theories on human subjects with the same condition. Level V evidence is considered the lowest because it is an option based on physiology principles and clinical expertise, which is not necessary supported by clinical research using real patients. Please see Table 6-4 for a review of research study design, Table 6-5 for a review of research terminology, and Figure 6-1 for more information on levels of evidence and locations of each level.

Finding Levels of Medical Evidence

Levels of evidence can be found in different places; therefore, it is important to know where each is found to increase the efficiency of your search. Basic science research (level V), case reports (level IV), and clinical studies (level II and III) can be found in basic medical science databases such as PubMed or Excerpta Medica Database (EMBASE). Typically, they are easily identified by the terms *case report* or *case series* found in their title. Randomized controlled trials (RCTs) (level I and II) can be found on Web sites such as Current Controlled Trials (www.controlled-trials.com). Systematic reviews and meta-analyses (level I) are found in databases such as the Cochrane Library, Database of Abstracts of Reviews of Effectiveness (DARE), or the Physiotherapy Evidence Database (PEDro). You and your student can also find level I evidence, including RCT, in basic medical science databases such as PubMed, but it is up to the reader to determine the level of evidence. Typically, level I evidence include the terms *systematic review* or *meta-analysis* in the title. Your student can identify RCT, either by the title or by the research design statement in the abstract. Students can search for level I evidence in PubMed by either using these terms in the search or by using the PubMed Clinical Queries Database, which can be can be accessed at http://www.ncbi.nlm.nih.gov/corehtml/query/static/clinical.shtml or via a link available on PubMed's homepage. The PubMed Clinical Queries Database automatically limits searches to systematic reviews, meta-analyses, and RCTs. Regardless of the database used students may need some guidance when first beginning.

Have your students first search the Cochrane Library, DARE databases, or another EBM database you are familiar with to see if they can find a systematic review or meta-analysis (level I evidence) publications that may contain relevant information for answering their clinical questions. If there is no level I evidence available (due to a lack of multiple randomized control trials), then they may need to use a more basic medical science database (such as PubMed) and see if they can find lower levels of evidence (levels II to V). You and your students should give preference to clinical trials (level II and III) over case reports (level IV), and case series (level IV) over basic research (level V). Using lower levels of evidence to answer clinical question(s) may be limited by the fact that evidence from a single study has less credibility than evidence from a systematic review, which synthesizes the results from several studies. Therefore, you and your students may need to draw your own conclusion based on information from several sources containing lower level evidence.

When looking for lower levels of evidence to answer clinical questions, it is important to understand that some types of research studies at this level are more useful than others based on their study design. For example, if you are trying to answer a clinical question regarding a diagnosis, prognosis, or the risk of harm, you would want to find evidence from cohort studies, which compare the results between 2 treatment groups.[12] If the question is regarding best treatment/therapy or prevention, then use studies with randomized control trials. Understanding that different research designs can better answer certain types of clinical questions will help you and your students

text continues on page 53

TABLE 6-4

RESEARCH STUDY DEFINITIONS AND EXAMPLES

RESEARCH TERM	DEFINITION	EXAMPLE
Basic science research	Research that tests theories at a basic level, typically a biological or physiological level, and is completed in a laboratory setting. The results may not have direct application to patient care.	Johns LD, Straub SJ, Howard SM. Variability in effective radiating area and output power of new ultrasound transducers at 3 MHz. *J Athl Train.* 2007;42(1):22-28.
Case report	An in-depth description of a patient's medical problem and the resolution.	Rich V, McCaslin E. Central cord syndrome in a high school wrestler: a case report. *J Athl Train.* 2006;41(3):341-344.
Case series	An in-depth description of several patients with similar medical conditions and their resolution are tracked over time.	Elias I, Dheer S, Zoga AC, Raikin SM, Morrison WB. Magnetic resonance imaging findings in bipartite medial cuneiform—a potential pitfall in diagnosis of midfoot injuries: a case series. *J Med Case Reports.* 2008;2:272. www.jmedicalcasereports.com/content/2/1/272. Accessed November 19, 2008.
		Pagnani M. Open capsular repair without bone block for recurrent anterior shoulder instability in patients with and without bony defects of the glenoid and/or humeral head. *Am J Sports Med.* 2008;36(9):1805-1812.
Cohort study	A research study in which a group of individuals sharing a common characteristic are followed for a period of time to determine the predominate issues.	Sugiura Y, Saito T, Sakuraba K, Sakuma K, Suzuki E. Strength deficits identified with concentric action of the hip extensors and eccentric action of the hamstrings predispose to hamstring injury in elite sprinters. *J Orthop Sports Phys Ther.* 2008;38(8):457-464.
		Neuman P, Englund M, Kostogiannis I, et al. Prevalence of tibiofemoral osteoarthitis 15 years after nonoperative treatment of anterior cruciate ligament injury: a prospective cohort study. *Am J Sports Med.* 2008;36(9):1717-1725.

continued

TABLE 6-4 continued

RESEARCH STUDY DEFINITIONS AND EXAMPLES

RESEARCH TERM	DEFINITION	EXAMPLE
Case control study	A research study in which each patient is matched with a similar patient (eg, demographics, disease state), who acts as his or her control.	Fox, J Docherty CL, Schrader J, Applegate T. Eccentric plantar-flexor torque deficits in participants with functional ankle instability. *J Athl Train.* 2008;43(1):51-54.
Clinical research	Research in which patients with an injury or disease are studied.	Bleakley CM, O'Connor S, Tully MA, et al. The PRICE study (protection rest ice compression elevation): design of a randomized controlled trial comparing standard versus cryokinetic ice application in the management of acute ankle sprain. *BMC Musculoskelet Disord.* 2007;8:125.
		Choi WJ, Lee JW, Han SH, Kim BS, Lee SK. Chronic lateral ankle instability: the effect of intra-articular lesions on clinical outcome. *Am J Sports Med.* 2008;36(11):2167-2172.
Meta-analysis	A research study in which the data from several research studies that address a similar research hypothesis are pooled together for analysis.	Grindstaff TL, Hammill RR, Tuzson AE. Neuromuscular control training programs and noncontact anterior cruciate ligament injury rates in female athletes: a numbers-needed-to-treat analysis. *J Athl Train.* 2006;41(4):450-456.
Randomized control trial	A research study in which patients are randomized in the intervention (there may be more than one) or control group.	Young MA, Cook JL, Purdam CR, Kiss ZS, Alfredson H. Eccentric decline squat protocol offers superior results at 12 months compared with traditional eccentric protocol for patellar tendinopathy in volleyball players. *Br J Sports Med.* 2005;39(2):102-105.
		Metz R, Verleisdonk E, Heijden G, et al. Acute achilles tendon rupture: minimally invasive surgery versus nonoperative treatment with immediate full weightbearing—a randomized controlled trial. *Am J Sports Med.* 2008;36:1688-1694.

continued

TABLE 6-4 continued

RESEARCH STUDY DEFINITIONS AND EXAMPLES

RESEARCH TERM	DEFINITION	EXAMPLE
Systematic review	A summary of the literature on a given topic. Specific guidelines are used to identify, appraise, select, and synthesize quality research relevant to the specific topic.	Pietrosimone BG, Brindstaff TL, Linens SW, Uczekaj E, Hertel J. A systematic review of prophylactic braces in the prevention of knee ligament injuries in collegiate football players. *J Athl Train.* 2008; 43(4):409-415.

TABLE 6-5

DEFINING COMMON EVIDENCE-BASED MEDICINE AND RESEARCH TERMS

TERM	DEFINITION
Confidence interval	A range of values that represent what expected future values should be with 95% confidence if the experiment was repeated. This indicates the strength of the data. Narrow confidence intervals are stronger than wide confidence intervals.
Control group	A group in the research study who does not receive the intervention. They are needed to determine how much change can be contributed by factors other than the intervention.
Diagnosis	The identification of something such as an injury, disease, or condition.
Gold standard	Accepted reference standard or diagnostic test for a particular injury, disease, or condition.
Likelihood ratio	Indicates the likelihood of a given test result in a patient with a injury, disease, or condition compared to the likelihood of the same result in a patient without the disease.
Prognosis	A prediction of how a patient's injury, disease, or condition will progress or the outcome of the injury, disease, or condition.
Randomization	A process that ensures every member of a population has an equal chance to be assigned to each group within a study.
Risk of harm	The amount of risk associated with a treatment.
Sensitivity	The probability of a positive test among those who have the injury, disease, or condition.
Specificity	The probability of a negative test among those who do not have the injury, disease, or condition.

TABLE 6-6

EVIDENCE-BASED MEDICINE PUBLIC DOMAIN DATABASES

DATABASE	WEB ADDRESS
British Medical Journal	http://clinicalevidence.bmj.com/ceweb/index.jsp
The Cochrane Collaboration	www.cochrane.org/
Physiotherapy Evidence Database (PEDro)	www.pedro.org.au/
PubMed	www.ncbi.nlm.nih.gov/sites/entrez/
Education Resources Information Center (ERIC)	www.eric.ed.gov/
US National Institutes of Health—ClinicalTrials.gov	http://clinicaltrials.gov/
Best Evidence Topics	www.bestbets.org
United Kingdom National Library for Health Clinical Knowledge Summaries	www.library.nhs.uk/default.aspx
Turning Research Into Practice (TRIP) database	www.tripdatabase.com/index.html
Best Evidence Medical Education (BEME)	www.bemecollaboration.org/beme/pages/index.html
Centre for Reviews and Dissemination	www.york.ac.uk/inst/crd/index.htm

find the appropriate level of evidence and will also help you limit your review to information that applies to your clinical question. Despite the fact that some types of research studies are better at answering certain types of clinical questions, it is important to find as much applicable evidence as possible. Using multiple sources reduces the chance that you make a decision based on the results of one investigation.

Teaching Students to Use Databases and Search Engines to Efficiently Find Medical Evidence

You may need to introduce your students to EBM databases and search engines. University libraries associated with medical schools may offer the greatest access to both subscription (available for a fee) and nonsubscription (public domain) EBM databases. Anyone who has access to the internet has access to free, nonsubscription databases. We have provided a listing of public domain databases (Table 6-6) as well as some subscription/membership/fee-based databases (Table 6-7). Even if your student has some knowledge of these databases, you should discuss the types of databases

TABLE 6-7

MEMBERSHIP OR SUBSCRIPTION DATABASES

DATABASE	WEB ADDRESS
OvidSP	http://gateway.ovid.com
EMBASE	www.embase.com
American College of Physicians (ACP) Journal Club	www.acpjc.org/index.html
British Medical Journal (BMJ) Clinical Evidence Current Evidence-Based Reviews	http://clinicalevidence.bmj.com/ceweb/conditions/conditions.jsp
EBM Online Journal	http://ebm.bmj.com
Essential Evidence Plus (formally known as InfoPOEMS/InfoRetriever)	www.essentialevidenceplus.com/index.cfm
PEPID	www.pepidonline.com

available in your particular setting. Access to databases will vary depending on the resources available at a particular clinical setting, just like available modalities differ between athletic training clinical settings. For example, a high school may only have access to the internet while a university with a medical school or a hospital may subscribe to OvidSP or EMBASE. It is important that students appreciate how the availability of databases and search engines may vary depending on their clinical setting, and influence their ability to locate evidence. In addition to using different databases, your students should also understand how to choose appropriate terms in their search for clinical evidence. Conducting an efficient and effective search is sometimes dependent on the search terms used and how those terms are used in conjunction with Boolean operating terms.

Boolean operating terms are words used to expand or limit your search. Some databases/search engines, such as PubMed and DARE, will allow users to limit and expand searches using *and, or,* and *not.* To demonstrate the use of Boolean operating terms, have your students do a simple exercise investigating tendonitis treatments. Have them search the PubMed database at www.pubmed.gov for the term *tendonitis.* The results of such a search would include all levels of evidence that contain any information on tendonitis. To expand the results to include instances where the term tendonosis might be used instead of tendonitis, have your student search for *tendonitis or tendonosis.* Now have your students search for the terms *tendonitis and treatment.* This search will limit the results to just those articles that discuss tendonitis and treatment. Other databases/search engines such as Google, Google Scholar, and those whose searches are powered by Google do not support Boolean terms. Therefore, your students will not be able to limit their search results by using Boolean terms *and,* or *not* nor expand their search using *or.* If *and* or *not* are included in the search terms, they either dropped or incorporated into the search terms by Google. To demonstrate this, have your students search Google Scholar for terms *tendonitis and treatment.* Google will ignore the *and* and the student should see a note at the top of the results screen indicating that *and* is not necessary. If they search *tendonitis not treatment*, the results will include articles with all 3 terms. Therefore, the use of Boolean terms will limit your search results in PubMed, but will not limit your results found with Google Scholar. To limit your search with Google Scholar you must use the Advanced Scholar Search settings, found to the right of the Google search bar.

You may also do well to consider the terms your students use in their searches. One method is to have them write down every search term and/or combination of search terms they used for their evidence search. After they have attempted a search and gathered the information, you and your students can review the quality (level of evidence) and quantity of information that they found. Does the information answer the clinical question? Was there too much information to review? The success of the search may depend on the search terms, or combination of search terms, used in the search. Using our previous search example for tendonitis, you can see that using similar terms or a combination of terms can either expand or limit your results. If the search did not yield the desired results or too much information was found, then new terms, or combination of terms, could be discussed. If the search was successful, were there certain terms, or combination of terms, that yielded better information than others? Again, a discussion regarding the search terms may help improve the efficiency of future searches.

Regardless of the search terms used, some searches may yield little applicable information. The results will vary depending on the amount of research published on a particular topic. Searches that yield little or no results can serve as a discussion point in helping your student understand that there might not always be evidence to answer his or her clinical questions, but he or she should always search.

Students need to develop both their skills at forming clinical questions and their ability to search different databases to gather applicable and valid information. As to not overwhelm novice students, you will want to limit their search assignments at first. For example, you may begin by asking the student to answer a clinical question about which you are familiar with the current evidence. You may also ask them to use a specific database (eg, PubMed or Cochrane) to search for information regarding the clinical question. After each search, you should discuss the outcomes of the search with your student, including the database used, the terms used, and the level of evidence found. Once the student has more experience finding evidence, you can encourage your student to develop his or her own clinical questions and search all available databases (such as those listed in Tables 6-6 or 6-7) using his or her own search terms. As mentioned previously, you could also consider using students to explore clinical questions that need to be investigated for your practice.[13]

Step 3: Teaching Students to Evaluate Evidence

Once students are able to locate the appropriate evidence, they must be able to critically evaluate its rigor and applicability for answering their clinical question. To evaluate the rigor of the evidence found, students will need to understand some of the basic terms found in EBM literature. The articles and Web site tutorials we suggested when introducing EBM to your students should explain terms such as *intervention*, *control*, *randomization*, *systematic review*, *meta-analysis*, *randomized control trials*, *gold standard*, *likelihood ratio*, *sensitivity*, and *specificity*. You can deepen your students understanding of these terms by revisiting the articles and EBM tutorials we have already suggested (see Tables 6-1 and 6-2) or the definitions of terms provided in Table 6-5. For a simple review of EBM terms, we recommend reading *Evidence-Based Medicine in a Nutshell: A Guide to Finding and Using the Best Evidence in Caring for Patients*.[10]

Students also need to understand it is necessary to evaluate all the evidence they find and determine the merit of each item. For example, when determining if a systematic review is valid, your students should ask if it is possible for useful research studies to be left out of the review. This is possible if you are using a systematic review that is several years old and does not include more recent research. Also, if the systematic review search was limited to the English language only, that means relevant studies published in another language would not be included. For clinical trials, students should determine if subjects were randomized to treatment groups and if treatment groups were similar at the start of the study. If treatment groups are not similar at the beginning, it is difficult to tell if changes were due to the treatment studied or group differences. Also, clinical trials that blind the subjects and clinicians who measure outcomes have less human bias and are considered superior to clinical trials that do not blind subjects and clinicians.

Besides evaluating the methods of systematic reviews and clinical trials, students also need to evaluate the results. First, they need to determine if the outcomes measure are important and valid means for assessing the intervention. If your clinical question is regarding how well diagnostic ultrasound detects rotator cuff tears but the researchers quantified how large the rotator cuff tendons were when viewed with diagnostic ultrasound, then the study results are not helpful at answering your clinical questions. Second, how large were the treatment effects? If a study demonstrated shoulder range of motion improved by 5 degrees more after a specific rehabilitation program for rotator cuff strains, would that be clinically significant? Probably not since most goniometric measurements have an error rate between 3 to 5 degrees; however, an increase of 10 degrees may be clinically significant. Just because a number is statically significant does not mean it has clinical significance. We have included a list (Table 6-8) of articles that you can use to help your students further understand how to critically evaluate different levels of evidence.

After students evaluate the rigor of the medical evidence, students need to decide if the evidence truly addresses their clinical question. Remember the first step to EBP is developing a specific clinical question using the PICO method, therefore each part of the clinical question needs to be addressed. Does the evidence apply to the specific patient population or problem addressed in their clinical question? In our previous example of a patient with a rotator cuff injury, the clinician would want to find information regarding adolescent athletes, not professional baseball pitchers. Is there evidence that analyzes the intervention in your student's clinical question? Does the evidence include the comparison treatment (eg, exercises versus surgery) in your student's clinical question? If so, what does the evidence say about the intervention and comparison in question? The clinician in our example would also want to locate evidence that compares the results of detecting a rotator cuff tear with diagnostic ultrasound compared to MRI. Once your student has determined the rigor and applicability of the evidence, he or she needs to decide how to apply that evidence to his or her clinical problem.

Step 4: Teaching Students to Apply Evidence to Clinical Decisions

Teaching students how to apply evidence to clinical decisions is the most important aspect of teaching EMP. In our rotator cuff example, the current evidence reveals an MRI and diagnostic ultrasound are comparable in detecting full thickness rotator cuff tears. Diagnostic ultrasound, however, is better at detecting partial tears and is also

TABLE 6-8

RESOURCES FOR USING MEDICAL LITERATURE

Bigby M. Evidence-based medicine in a nutshell: a guide to finding and using the best evidence in caring for patients. *Arch Dermatol.* 1998;134(9):1609-1618.

Guyatt GH, Sackett DL, Cook DJ. Users' guides to the medical literature. II. How to use an article about therapy or prevention. B. What were the results and will they help me in caring for my patients? Evidence-Based Medicine Working Group. *JAMA.* 1994;271(1):59-63.

Jaeschke R, Guyatt G, Sackett DL. Users' guides to the medical literature. III. How to use an article about a diagnostic test. A. Are the results of the study valid? Evidence-Based Medicine Working Group. *JAMA.* 1994;271:389-391.

Oxman AD, Sackett DL, Guyatt GH. Users' guides to the medical literature. I. How to get started. Evidence-Based Medicine Working Group. *JAMA.* 1993;3(17):2093-2095.

more cost effective.[6] If the patient wants to compete in collegiate sports, it may be important to the patient to detect a partial tear. Therefore, ultrasound could be used based on the evidence. However, real patient cases are often more complicated than the simulations or case studies that may be presented in the classroom. It is important for your student to consider the evidence found as well as any clinical experience he or she might have when providing patient care. In addition, personalities of those involved, such as the patient, coach, and parents (if the patient is a minor), may also influence your student's diagnosis and treatment. For example, the patient's parent may object to driving their son to the diagnostic ultrasound facility because it is in another town further away than the local MRI imaging center. Because clinical cases can be more complex, students need to understand the application of clinical evidence may not be as straight forward as the application to hypothetical simulations or case studies. Some clinicians have developed evidence appraisal checklists to use to evaluate and determine when evidence should be used for a particular patient's problem.[11] Please see Table 6-9 for an example. For additional appraisal checklists, please see the EBM tools on the Centre for Evidence-Based Medicine website at www.cebm.net.

Step 5: Teaching Students How to Evaluate Their Evidence-Based Practice

EBP is about using the most current and relevant medical evidence to guide your clinical practice. In order for this to occur, you and your students need to reflect on the use of the evidence to address clinical problems. To assist reflection and evaluate your ATSs' EBP, together you and your students should evaluate the effectiveness of the steps taken and seek ways to improve future patient care. A self-evaluation regarding whether you and your students are answering answerable questions, finding the best evidence, critically evaluating the evidence for its validity and potential usefulness, integrating critical appraisal with clinical expertise and applying the result in clinical practice, and changing clinical practice behavior is essential.[2]

TABLE 6-9

EXAMPLE APPRAISAL CHECKLIST

Citation:		
Patient/Problem:		Notes:
	Did the study use subjects similar (eg, gender, age, activity level) to your patient?	
	Were subjects randomized and blinded?	
	Were the groups similar (eg, demographic, pre-treatment values) at the start of the study?	
Intervention:		
	Was the intervention assessed using meaningful outcome measures?	
Comparison:		
	Was a comparison group used? Was the intervention group compared to a control group?	
Outcomes:		
	What were the outcome results?	
	How large was the treatment effect?	
	Do the results apply to your patient?	
	Is your patient similar to those in the study?	
	Is the treatment feasible in your setting?	
	Do you and your patient have a clear assessment of his or her values and preferences?	
	Are your patient's values met by this treatment and its consequences?	
	Will the potential benefits of the treatment outweigh any harm or risk?	

Some specific questions you and your student might ask would be:

- Did we ask a well-formed clinical question?
- Did we have a method to save our clinical question to answer at a later time?
- Did we use the best sources of information for our discipline?
- Were we more efficient with our current search compared to previous searches?
- Did we use the best search terms, or combination of search terms, in our search?
- Are we critically appraising the evidence that we found before we used it?
- Were we able to integrate the evidence into our current clinical practice?
- Will we change our clinical practice and future patient care based on the evidence we have found and implemented?
- Could we have improved this process in any way?

You and your students should discuss your answers to these questions. You should also address any barriers to EBP, such as database and search engine access, or a general lack of evidence for your current patient problem. It is important to impress on your student that this self-evaluation process is part of improving EBP. Reflecting on the EBP experience will help improve your ability to find and apply EBM to your next clinical problem.

SUMMARY

For your ATSs to be effective clinicians and improve patient outcomes, it is important to learn how to adapt clinical practice as new evidence becomes available. EBP requires clinicians to be lifelong learners who are consumers of research and apply it to their clinical practice. However, your students need to appreciate the benefits and limitations of the new evidence.[11] Depending on your setting and patient population, not all evidence will be applicable to your practice. Even so, it is still important for you to model EBP behaviors for your students. You play an important role in influencing student's future use of EBP to help ensure that they can provide quality patient care. Quite simply, as an ACI, you play a pivotal role in influencing how future athletic trainers practice since students develop their attitudes and behaviors toward EBP based on their clinical experiences.

REFLECTION QUESTIONS

- Describe the difference between evidence-based medicine and evidence based practice.
- List some databases that you will use to investigate evidence and the level(s) of evidence you will find in those databases.
- Plan 2 assignments for your students that will assist them in understanding the 5 steps of EBM.
- Develop a plan in which you will incorporate EBP into you and your students' clinical practice. How will you save clinical questions for searches at a later time? When will you perform searches and review the results of those searches?

REFERENCES

1. Evidence-Based Medicine Working Group. Evidence-based medicine: a new approach to teaching the practice of medicine. *JAMA*. 1992;268(17):2420-2425.
2. Sackett DL, Straus SE, Richardson WS, Rosenberg W, Haynes RB. *Evidence-Based Medicine: How to Practice and Teach EBM*. 3rd ed. Edinburgh, Scotland: Elsevier Chruchill Livingtonstone; 2005.
3. Steves R, Hootman JM. Evidence-based medicine: what is it and how does it apply to athletic training? *J Athl Train*. 2004;39(1):83-87.
4. Nicholson LJ, Warde CM, Boker JR. Faculty training in evidence-based medicine: improving evidence acquisition and critical appraisal. *J Contin Educ Health Prof*. 2007;27(1):28-33.
5. Hurwitz SR, Slawson D, Shaughnessy A. Orthopaedic information mastery: applying evidence-based information tools to improve patient outcomes while saving orthopaedists' time. *J Bone Joint Surg Am*. 2000;82(6):888-894.
6. Dinnes J, Loveman E, McIntyre L, Waugh N. The effectiveness of diagnostic tests for the assessment of shoulder pain due to soft tissue disorders: a systematic review. *Health Technol Assess*. 2003;7(29): iii, 1-166.
7. Yew KS, Reid A. Teaching evidence-based medicine skills: an exploratory study of residency graduates' practice habits. *Fam Med*. 2008;40(1):24-31.
8. Coomarasamy A, Khan KS. What is the evidence that postgraduate teaching in evidence based medicine changes anything? A systematic review. *BMJ*. 2004;329(7473):1017.
9. Wyer PC, Keitz S, Hatala R, et al. Tips for learning and teaching evidence-based medicine: introduction to the series. *CMAJ*. 2004;171(4):347-348.
10. Bigby M. Evidence-based medicine in a nutshell: a guide to finding and using the best evidence in caring for patients. *Arch Dermatol*. 1998;134(12):1609-18.
11. Hazlett CB. Teaching evidence-based medicine. *Hong Kong Med J*. 1998;4(2):183-190.
12. Levine M, Walter S, Lee H, et al. Users' guides to the medical literature. IV. How to use an article about harm. Evidence-Based Medicine Working Group. *JAMA*. 1994;271(20):1615-1619.
13. Kelly EK, Hunley AL, Wegner JL, et al. Evidence-based nursing: making changes in the clinical practice through the collaboration of nursing students and practicing nurses. *Appl Nurs Res*. 2005;18(4):229-231.

7

Initial and Continuing Approved Clinical Instructor Training

Thomas G. Weidner, PhD, ATC, FNATA

Because excellent clinical skills do not guarantee expertise as a clinical instructor, the profession of athletic training is making a concerted effort to provide training and development for clinical instructors. Accordingly, Standards for an Accredited Educational Program for the Athletic Trainer includes standards regarding Clinical Instructor Educators (CIEs) and Approved Clinical Instructors (ACIs).[1] Table 7-1 shows the qualifications and responsibilities of CIEs and ACIs.[1]

If more than one individual is designated as the CIE for the educational program, then at least one of those individuals must be a BOC credentialed athletic trainer.[1] Ideally, all or most clinicians associated with an athletic training educational program (ATEP) will complete ACI training for the role of clinical instructor.

ACI training is specific to the ATEP. Thus, individuals who complete the training become ACIs for that program only. If an individual relocates or chooses to be an ACI for additional ATEPs, s/he must complete training for each one, although the CIE may reduce this training to program/institution-specific policies, procedures, and clinical education requirements (see initial ACI training section).

Clearly, an ACI should improve both the quality and consistency of clinical education for each athletic training student in the ATEP. Essentially, the CIE is responsible for implementing the CAATE standards regarding training/retraining the ACIs for the ATEP, and the ACIs are responsible for carrying out clinical education for the ATEP. This chapter will address the content areas required for initial ACI training, recommend content for initial ACI training and continuing training, suggest delivery strategies for such training, and overview documentation regarding this training. Lastly, a list of incentives for attracting and retaining ACIs will be considered.

TABLE 7-1

QUALIFICATIONS AND RESPONSIBILITIES OF CIES AND ACIS

CIE QUALIFICATIONS

Approval of ATEP

Board of Certification credential (3 year minimum)

Institutional authorization to oversee ACI training

Knowledge of content areas required for ACI training

CIE RESPONSIBILITIES

Train and retrain ACIs for the ATEP

ACI QUALIFICATIONS

Professional training from ATEP

Professional credential in health care profession as defined by American Medical Association or American Osteopathic Association (eg, physical therapist, physician assistant, EMT)

Cannot be currently a student within the ATEP

ACI RESPONSIBILITIES

Instruction and/or evaluation of Athletic Training Educational Competencies

Assessment of athletic training students' clinical proficiencies

Regular communication with appropriate ATEP administrator

Understanding of and compliance with the policies and procedures of the ATEP

CONTENT FOR INITIAL APPROVED CLINICAL INSTRUCTOR TRAINING

Accreditation standards[1] for initial ACI training stipulate the following content areas:

- Learning styles and instructional skills
- Review of the Athletic Training Educational Competencies
- Evaluation of student performance and feedback
- Instructional skills of supervision, mentoring, and administration
- Program/institution-specific policies, procedures, and clinical education requirements
- Legal and ethical behaviors
- Communication skills
- Appropriate interpersonal relationships
- Appropriate clinical skills and knowledge

Table 7-2 lists appropriate topics/essential messages for each of the required content areas, as well as additional content areas and associated topics/essential messages for initial ACI training. The CIE develops the essential messages for each of these areas to

text continues on page 67

TABLE 7-2

CONTENT AREAS AND ASSOCIATED POTENTIAL TOPICS/ ESSENTIAL MESSAGES FOR INITIAL ACI TRAINING

REQUIRED CONTENT AREAS

1. Learning styles and instructional skills

- Collaborate with the program director and/or clinical education coordinator to plan learning experiences.

- Implement, facilitate, and evaluate planned learning experiences with athletic training students.

- Understand the athletic training students' academic curriculum, level of didactic preparation, and current level of performance relative to the goals of the clinical education experience.

- Take advantage of teachable moments during planned and unplanned learning experiences by instructing skills or content that is meaningful and immediately applicable.

- Employ a variety of teaching styles to meet individual athletic training students' needs.

- Help athletic training students' progress toward meeting the goals and objectives of the clinical experience as assigned by the program director and/or clinical education coordinator.

- Modify learning experiences based on the athletic training students' strengths and weaknesses.

- Create learning opportunities that actively engage athletic training students in the clinical setting and that promote problem solving and critical thinking.

- Encourage self-directed learning activities for the athletic training students when appropriate.

- Perform regular self-appraisal of teaching methods and effectiveness.

- Be enthusiastic about teaching athletic training students.

- Communicate complicated/detailed concepts in terms that students can understand based on their level of progression within the athletic training education program.

- Encourage athletic training students to engage in self-directed learning as a means of establishing lifelong learning practices of inquiry and clinical problem solving.

2. Review of the Athletic Training Educational Competencies

- Recognize the 12 content areas around which curriculum and clinical education are established.

- Understand the classifications/distinctions of cognitive and psychomotor competencies, foundations of professional practice, and clinical proficiencies.

- Understand how to implement "learning over time" as a component of students' clinical education (eg, previous coursework and clinical experiences completed, objectives for current clinical rotation).

- Include skills that reflect evidenced-based knowledge and practice in athletic training.

continued

TABLE 7-2 continued

CONTENT AREAS AND ASSOCIATED POTENTIAL TOPICS/ ESSENTIAL MESSAGES FOR INITIAL ACI TRAINING

REQUIRED CONTENT AREAS

3. Evaluation of student performance and feedback

- Note the athletic training students' knowledge, skills, and behaviors as they relate to the specific goals and objectives of their clinical experience.

- Communicate with the Program Director and/or Clinical Education Coordinator regarding implementing and/or clarifying the ATEP's performance evaluation instruments.

- Record student progress based on performance criteria established by the ATEP and identify areas of competence as well as areas that require improvement.

- Approach the evaluation process as constructive and educational.

- Communicate with the Program Director and/or Clinical Education Coordinator in a timely manner when an athletic training student needs remediation. The ACI and athletic training students participate in formative (ie, on-going specific feedback) and summative (ie, general overall performance feedback) evaluations.

4. Supervision, mentoring, and administration

- Directly supervise athletic training students during formal acquisition, practice, and evaluation of the Entry-Level Athletic Training Clinical Proficiencies.

- Intervene on behalf of the athlete/patient when the athletic training student is putting the athlete/patient at risk or harm.

- Encourage athletic training students to arrive at clinical decisions on their own according to their level of education and clinical experience.

- Apply the clinical education policies, procedures, and expectations of the ATEP.

- Present clear performance expectations to athletic training students at the beginning and throughout the learning experience.

- Inform athletic training students of relevant policies and procedures of the clinical setting.

- Provide feedback to athletic training students from information acquired from direct observation, discussion with others, and review of athlete/patient documentation.

- Treat the athletic training students' presence as educational and not as a means for providing medical coverage.

- Complete athletic training students' evaluation forms requested for the ATEP in a timely fashion.

- Provide the Program Director and/or Clinical Education Coordinator with requested materials as required for the accreditation process.

- Collaborate with athletic training students to arrange quality clinical education experiences that are compatible with the students' academic schedules.

continued

TABLE 7-2 continued

CONTENT AREAS AND ASSOCIATED POTENTIAL TOPICS/ ESSENTIAL MESSAGES FOR INITIAL ACI TRAINING

REQUIRED CONTENT AREAS

5. Program/institution-specific policies, procedures, and clinical education requirements

- Mission and expectations of the ATEP.

- Criteria for retention in the ATEP.

- Clinical supervision responsibilities and evaluation of clinical experiences.

- Clinical education policies (eg, blood borne pathogens, therapeutic modalities and therapeutic rehabilitation/exercise, infectious illness).

- Technical standards for admission and retention in the ATEP.

- Dress code expectations.

- CAATE clinical education terminology.

- Curricula.

6. Legal and ethical behaviors

- Hold the appropriate credential BOC certification and state license, registration, certification, or exemption, if applicable as required by the state in which the individual provides athletic training services.

- Provide athletic training services that are defined by the *Role Delineation Study* and within the scope of the respective state practice act (if applicable).

- Provide athletic training services that are consistent with state and federal legislation (eg, equal opportunity and affirmative action policies, ADA, HIPAA, and FERPA).

- Demonstrate ethical behavior as defined by the NATA *Code of Ethics* and the BOC *Standards of Professional Practice*.

7. Communication skills

- Communicate with the Program Director and/or Clinical Education Coordinator regarding athletic training students' progress toward clinical education goals at regularly scheduled intervals determined by the athletic training education program.

- Use appropriate forms of verbal and written communication clearly and concisely with athletic training students.

- Provide appropriately timed and constructive formative and summative feedback to athletic training students.

- Facilitate communication with athletic training students through open-ended questions and directed problem solving.

- Ensure time for on-going professional discussions with athletic training students in the clinical setting.

- Communicate with athletic training students in a nonconfrontational and positive manner.

- Receive and respond to feedback from the Program Director, Clinical Education Coordinator, and athletic training students.

continued

TABLE 7-2 continued

CONTENT AREAS AND ASSOCIATED POTENTIAL TOPICS/ ESSENTIAL MESSAGES FOR INITIAL ACI TRAINING

REQUIRED CONTENT AREAS

8. Appropriate interpersonal relationships

- Form appropriate and professional relationships with athletic training students.
- Model appropriate and professional interpersonal relationships when interacting with athletic training students, colleagues, patients/athletes, and administrators.
- Appropriately advocate athletic training students when interacting with colleagues, patients/athletes, and administrators.
- Be a positive role model and/or mentor for athletic training students.
- Demonstrate respect for gender, racial, ethnic, religious, and individual differences when interacting with people.
- Maintain an open and approachable demeanor to athletic training students when working in the clinical setting.

9. Appropriate clinical skills and knowledge

- Capable of teaching and evaluating the clinical proficiencies that are particular to their setting or environment.
- Knowledge and skills are current and support care decisions based on science and evidence-based practice.
- Maintain clinical skills and knowledge through participation in continuing education programs.

SUGGESTED CONTENT AREAS

1. Roles/responsibilities of the clinical education setting

- Active and stimulating learning environment.
- Meets specific objectives of the educational program and the individual student.
- Variety of learning experiences available to students.
- Administrative interest in and support of athletic training clinical education.
- Adequate number of clinical instructors to provide a good educational experience.
- Clinical instructor is responsible for coordinating student assignments and activities.

2. One-minute preceptor

- Steps of OMP.
- Fostering effective and efficient teaching.
- Steps for integrating into clinical teaching.

continued

TABLE 7-2 continued

CONTENT AREAS AND ASSOCIATED POTENTIAL TOPICS/ ESSENTIAL MESSAGES FOR INITIAL ACI TRAINING

SUGGESTED CONTENT AREAS

3. Challenges for the ACI

- Student confidence level.
- Student conflict with instructors, staff, and coaches.
- Inappropriate student social interaction.
- Student time management

use in training their future ACIs. In the process, teaching strategies (see section later in this chapter) for presenting these essential messages during ACI training needs to be considered. See Appendix H for a worksheet designed to guide the CIE in developing the content/essential messages and teaching strategies for initial ACI training. This textbook should serve as a starting point for information and insights to complete the worksheet; also see Appendix A for a listing of helpful online clinical teaching resources. There is no hour requirement for initial ACI training.

CONTINUING APPROVED CLINICAL INSTRUCTOR TRAINING

Accreditation standards require that ACIs be trained/retrained by the institution's CIE at least once every 3 years.[1] As with initial ACI training, there is no specific hour requirement for this training. As well, there are no required content areas for such training. The CIE could consider needed topics for continuing ACI training through the following strategies:

- Conversing with ACIs
- Observing ACIs as they interact with students in the clinical setting
- Reviewing student evaluations of ACIs
- ACI self-assessing strengths/weaknesses (see Appendix C)

With this information, the ACI can develop an annual professional development plan that consists of goals, action steps, and a timeline for completion. Additional assessment information to consider for developing this plan could be provided through the routine student evaluations of the ACI (see Appendix B). Also, the CIE and/or a peer ACI can provide meaningful input through occasionally evaluating the ACI (see Appendix B).

In addition to continuing emphasis on the content areas presented in Table 7-2, other potential topics could include the following:

- Evaluating clinical proficiencies
- Challenges in clinical education

- Professional development
- Interdisciplinary teamwork
- Effective clinical teaching
- Evidence-based practice and clinical education
- The One-Minute Preceptor
- Integrating the student into a busy clinical practice
- Clinical outcomes assessment and clinical education

STRATEGIES FOR DELIVERING INITIAL AND CONTINUING APPROVED CLINICAL INSTRUCTOR TRAINING

Provided below are several suggestions to consider as you develop and adapt your own approach to effective ACI training. Use these ideas to trigger other creative strategies. Certainly, the CIE for each ATEP will have a multitude of factors unique to the situation/institution when it comes to delivering and designing ACI training.

The more conventional model for delivering ACI training is in face-to-face sessions. One such approach is to conduct a several hour session in one block of time. Although efficient, it may be exceedingly difficult to get everyone together for a larger block of time. In that case, consider conducting several smaller sessions, or "modules," staggered over a 2- to 3-month period. An additional advantage of such an approach is that training content can be implemented into clinical teaching between sessions and then reflected upon at the next training session before additional training is delivered. From a teaching standpoint, this is likely a stronger approach for delivering face-to-face training.

Another model to consider is online training. As in the face-to-face training conducted over several smaller sessions, training content can be delivered as modules, and then implemented and reflected upon before additional training is completed. Continuing ACI training could also be designed as individual learning modules. An ACI could be instructed to complete a certain number of these modules from a menu of such modules based on the interests/needs of the ACI. Certainly, an additional advantage of the online training model is that training can be completed at the convenience of the busy professional. This may prove to be an important way to attract and retain ACIs.

There are numerous approaches for designing ACI training, depending upon the delivery model used. Teaching and learning offices/centers can be very helpful in this process. Consider, for instance, incorporating skits into your ACI training. At first, the skit could be created and led by the CIE. Afterwards, to reinforce learning, the training participants could create and act their own skit. Concepts that could lend themselves very nicely to skits include supervision of clinical education versus clinical experience, and clinical proficiency evaluation. Video segments could also be created and similarly utilized. Consider organizing expert ACI panel discussions covering a variety of challenges that may confront the ACI, and strategies for managing them. See the list on the next page for examples of such challenges. ACI training participants should also weigh-in regarding their own insights for managing the situations as well as posing other challenges that they may have experienced.

CHALLENGES IN CLINICAL EDUCATION

Student Related

Behavior

1. *Motivation level:* A junior athletic training student has just completed a practicum at a local high school that she did not particularly enjoy because it was not in line with her career goals. The student is now returning to campus to gain clinical experience with off-season soccer. The student is very unenthusiastic about the clinical assignment and feels "shafted" because it is not an in-season sport. The academic year is drawing to a close and the student just wants to go home for the summer.

   o What can you as the student's ACI do to keep the student motivated?

   o What teaching techniques/strategies might you use to stimulate the student's interest?

2. *Confidence level:* A first semester athletic training student does not appear to be progressing in the clinical proficiencies at the same rate as his classmates. The student is performing poorly on practical exams but is doing extremely well on written exams. You have noticed that the student is very apprehensive in the clinical environment and many of the student athletes/patients will not approach him for assistance.

   o What can you as the student's ACI do to assist in improving confidence?

   o What techniques might you use to make the student feel more comfortable in the clinical setting?

3. *Conflict with instructors, staff, and coaches:* A senior athletic training student has successfully completed all of the clinical proficiencies required for the athletic training program. The student is in her last semester in the program and is preparing to take the BOC exam in April. She is feeling very confident. Her clinical assignment this spring is working with the men's and women's track and field teams. At practice one day she inappropriately questions your decision regarding the status of a female distance runner in front of the athlete and the coach.

   o How do you handle this unprofessional act by the student?

   o What is the goal/purpose that directs your reaction?

Social Interaction

1. *Peers:* Two of your top senior students have been assigned to a clinical experience with in-season football. You have encouraged them both to strengthen their leadership skills and be role models for the younger students.

   One of the senior students, John, thought the students would work together better if they were a "tight knit group." John planned a social outing for the group that involved playing drinking games. John got very drunk and started talking "trash" about the other senior athletic training student, Jan, whom he did not invite to the social gathering. The underclassmen no longer respect John after this event.

   Jan decided to make a real effort at developing her leadership skills. She was very organized and planned daily duties for the underclassmen working with football. However, Jan was too busy telling people what to do instead of helping them do it. The underclassmen started to resent her.

As the ACI, you notice a great deal of tension among the group of students. You also notice that daily assignments are not being completed.

○ What is your plan of action for handling this dysfunctional group?

2. *Patients:* One busy afternoon in the athletic training room, you overhear an inappropriate conversation between an athletic training student and an athlete. They are discussing a party they attended over the weekend and planning a date for the following weekend. The athletic training student and the athlete are very flirtatious with one another in the athletic training room and at the practice venue.

○ What are your steps for resolving this inappropriate situation?

Time Management Related

1. *Supervision and instruction:* It is the end of the regular season and your team is preparing for the conference tournament. You are receiving a lot of heat from the coaching staff to "fix" two of the key players for tournament action. Your stress level is through the roof and your day is planned around multiple rehabilitation sessions and practice. On top of your work responsibilities, your spouse is out of town on business and you have to taxi your kids around.

○ How can you ensure that your athletic training student will not be neglected in this stressful environment?

2. *Athletic training student time management:* You have noticed that your athletic training student is more stressed than normal. The student seems to be forgetting routine tasks and seems unfocused. You are informed through a regular staff meeting that this particular student is having difficulty in one of the required athletic training courses.

○ What are your steps for helping to resolve this situation?

Another helpful tool in designing ACI training is a clinical education reference handbook that presents relevant policies and procedures regarding clinical education in your ATEP. This informational piece could be printed in hardcopy and/or posted online. Sample contents of such a handbook could include the following:

- Mission of the ATEP
- Expectations of the ATEP
- Criteria for retention in the ATEP
- Clinical experience expectations and classroom responsibilities
- Clinical supervision
- Evaluation of clinical experiences

Sample appendices:

- Emergency Action Plan Orientation Checklist
- Blood Borne Pathogens Policy
- Therapeutic Modalities and Therapeutic Rehabilitation/Exercise Policy
- Technical Standards for Admission and Retention Considerations
- Dress Code Expectations
- CAATE Clinical Education Terminology
- Infectious Illness Policy
- Curricula

DOCUMENTING INITIAL AND CONTINUING APPROVED CLINICAL INSTRUCTOR TRAINING

Document the following upon completion of initial and/or continuing ACI training:

- Completion date of initial and continuing training
- Agenda/content
- Contact hours
- Names and BOC certification numbers of CIEs and participants
- Place of employment of participants

Consider placing a record online regarding your ACIs' retraining status so that you and the ACIs can monitor training requirements. As well, a formal letter can serve to both thank the ACI for completing training and to verify that training has been completed. In this letter, also indicate the number of CEUs for which the ACI is elgible. This can be determined as follows:

- For the ACI training, one CEU is awarded to the ACI participant per contact hour
- An ACI who has taken the training from a CIE who has received approval as a BOC CEU provider can count CEUs in Category A (up to 75 CEUs)
- If the ACI training is given by a CIE who is a nonapproved provider, the ACI would count the CEUs in Category D (up to 20 CEUs)
- A CIE who conducts an ACI training is awarded 10 CEUs under Category B as a presenter. If the material is different, a CIE can count 10 CEUs per training/presentation

At this point it would also be helpful to have your new ACI(s) complete a specifically designed evaluation survey regarding the initial/continuing ACI training. Use this information to improve current training and to develop further training.

INCENTIVES FOR SERVING AS AN APPROVED CLINICAL INSTRUCTOR

In that ACIs are busy health care professionals who juggle a multitude of roles, it is important to recognize their efforts in serving as an ACI in your ATEP. Listed below are some examples of professional courtesy incentives that you can use to recognize your ACIs' contributions.

- List names of ACIs in alumni newsletters
- Create an Outstanding ACI Award to recognize exemplary performance (notify supervisors and administrators)
- Invite to social and professional functions of the ATEP
- Provide complimentary textbooks, journal subscriptions, etc
- Send thank you notes (particulary handwritten)
- Send thank you letters, which are copied to supervisors and administrators
- Provide small honorariums (as feasible)
- Recognize with adjunct professor status (which may include library privileges, parking, etc)

- Orient students that the time the ACI is giving them warrants their genuine appreciation

- Provide complimentary tickets to attend athletic events (or other events on campus)

REFERENCE

1. Commission on Accreditation of Athletic Training Education. *Standards for the Accreditation of Entry Level Educational Programs for the Athletic Trainer.* Round Rock, TX: Author; 2006.

SECTION II

STRATEGIES FOR EFFECTIVE TEACHING AND LEARNING IN THE CLINICAL SETTING

8

See One, Do One, Teach One
Peer-Assisted Learning in the Clinical Setting

Jolene M. Henning, EdD, ATC, LAT and Thomas G. Weidner, PhD, ATC, FNATA

Athletic training professional preparation has been rapidly evolving over the past 15 years. It has progressed away from loosely structured internship routes to highly structured accredited programs. Standards[1] established for these accredited programs place a great deal of emphasis on quality clinical education, including a vast array of clinical skills. Consequently, as an Approved Clinical Instructor (ACI), you are charged with greater responsibility for ensuring that students learn and master a cadre of clinical skills. You are probably already encountering significant role strain as you attempt to balance patient care and student education.[2] Coupled with this increase in educational responsibilities is the accreditation standard that regulates the amount of clinical hours students can obtain thus requiring you to implement creative strategies for fostering quality clinical education in a limited amount of time.[3] This will undoubtedly require a team approach to clinical education that not only includes you as a supervisor but also capitalizing on athletic training students (ATSs) for teaching/tutoring, providing feedback, and mentoring their peers. To this end, we suggest that peer-assisted learning (PAL) be implemented in clinical education as a means to supplement your role as the ACI.[4] Throughout this chapter we will define PAL and its benefits as well as illustrate its application in the clinical education setting.

DEFINITION OF PEER-ASSISTED LEARNING

PAL is conceptualized in the literature as a multi-faceted model of student interactions in which multiple peers benefit from the exchange.[5,6] To further define PAL, we will explore each aspect of the term. ATS peers can include students in the same level of the ATEP or those in upper or lower levels of the program. The key with any type of PAL or any level of peer is that all parties stand to benefit from the interaction. Further, learning can be defined as to gain knowledge, understanding, or skill through instruction or experience.[6] PAL includes peer teaching and learning, peer assessment, peer mentoring, and peer leadership. Therefore, PAL is the act or process of gaining knowledge, understanding, or skill in athletic training from students that are either at different or equivalent academic/experiential levels.[4]

PAL has not only been demonstrated to reduce demands on you as an ACI, but to also improve the overall clinical experiences for students.[7] PAL should never be used to replace your role as the ACI in providing initial instruction, evaluation, supervision, and role modeling.[4] Rather, you can use PAL to encourage students to practice and reinforce clinical skills[8] and professional behaviors.

Peer Teaching and Learning

You are probably familiar with the old adage "see one, do one, teach one." This phrase is a good descriptor for how PAL can be used in the process of learning over time where students learn a skill from an ACI, practice it on a patient, and then teach a peer. More formally, peer teaching is defined as a student-centered approach to instruction and can simply be defined as the process of students teaching their peers.[9] Peer learning is defined as acquiring knowledge from a peer through study, experience, observation, or teaching.[10]

Students in the roles of "teacher" and "learner" both stand to benefit from the educational interaction in the clinical setting.[5,8,11,12] See Table 8-1 for the mutual benefits experienced by students during peer teaching and learning encounters.

Research regarding PAL in entry-level athletic training professional preparation has clearly revealed its prevalence and effectiveness. In surveying undergraduate students at the Athletic Training Student Seminar at the National Athletic Trainers' Association 2002 Annual Meeting and Clinical Symposia, 66% of the students reported that they practice a moderate to high amount of their clinical skills with other ATS.[3] Very importantly, 60% of these students reported feeling less anxious when performing clinical skills on patients in front of other ATS compared to in front of their ACIs.[3] Certainly, this can have important ramifications for improving learning for your ATS. Another study[8] actually provided evidence for the use of intentional, formal PAL on the performance of psychomotor skills. Fifty-one undergraduate students were examined regarding their pre/post-test performance scores (number of correct skills) and the amount of time to complete the skills in 3 categories of hand/wrist orthopedic evaluation psychomotor skills. Subjects were assigned to either a peer tutor or an ACI review group. Students who practiced their skills with a peer tutor performed psychomotor skills related to the orthopedic assessment of the wrist and hand as competently as those students who practiced their skills with an ACI. It appears that PAL can be a valuable adjunct during clinical education. We recommend that PAL not only be encouraged, but that time should be purposefully designated in the clinical setting for students to practice skills with their peers, especially without the anxiety of formal evaluation.

Implementing Peer Teaching and Learning

You have probably observed students naturally teaching and learning from one another in the clinical setting but with a little planning, you can maximize on this natural tendency and foster deeper learning and understanding in your students.

An obvious component for facilitating peer teaching and learning, as well as the other forms of PAL, is that there must be more than one ATS assigned to you as the ACI at one time. Peer teaching and learning is effective among students of the same level

TABLE 8-1

BENEFITS OF PEER TEACHING AND LEARNING

BENEFITS FOR THE "PEER TEACHER"

- Improved study habits[11]
- Better attitudes toward the subject matter[11]
- Beneficial review of clinical concepts[13]
- Improved communication skills[13]
- Increased self-confidence[13]

BENEFITS FOR THE "PEER LEARNER"

- Reinforced self-confidence[14]
- Enhanced clinical skills and acquisition of new information[14]
- Reinforced previously learned information and techniques[14]
- Improved ability to accept feedback[14]
- Decreased stress when practicing skills with peers[15]

MUTUAL BENEFITS

- Improved psychomotor test scores[16]
- Improved overall clinical knowledge[16]
- Improved critical thinking skills[17]
- Less dependence on clinical instructor[17]
- Sense of increased responsibility and independence in the clinical setting[18]
- Enhanced collaborative approach to patient care[18]
- Decreased anxiety in new clinical situations[15]

as well as between different levels of students. For example, junior students can learn from each other while also teaching sophomores. Consider with your program's clinical education coordinator ways that you can supervise multiple students in one rotation. As well, you might also consider having students reflect on their peer teaching and learning experiences in their journals or update reports. Likely, this will reinforce the value and benefits of engaging in peer teaching and learning activities and foster continued participation. One other way to foster peer teaching and learning might be through serving as peer lab teachers alongside the ACI in a variety of athletic training courses.

PEER LEADERSHIP

Thinking back to your experiences as an ATS, you can probably recall situations when you were asked to assume a leadership role as the "head" or "lead" student for

TABLE 8-2

BENEFITS OF PEER LEADERSHIP

BENEFITS FOR ATHLETIC TRAINING STUDENTS

- Increased practical knowledge of how to prioritize patient care[21]
- Improved ability to multitask[21]
- Enhanced organizational skills[21]
- Gained a more realistic understanding of the real world role as health care providers[21]
- Increased sense of self-awareness regarding their clinical skills[22]
- Increased self-confidence in the ability to supervise a colleague[22]

BENEFITS FOR APPROVED CLINICAL INSTRUCTORS

- Increased time available for clinical teaching[17]

a team as an upper classman. This is still a common practice in ATEPs today and can lead to the development of positive leadership characteristics. Multiple definitions and descriptions exist for the complex concept of leadership.[19] For the purpose of this chapter, peer leadership is defined as a more experienced student giving directions/ guidance or delegating tasks to a less experienced peer in the clinical setting.

Certainly with this type of student leadership role is the implied responsibility for students to delegate tasks to their peers as well as being proactive in planning and multitasking in the clinical environment.[20] This is not to imply that students with leadership roles should take the place of a credentialed ACI. On the contrary, more experienced students can assist the ACI with the delegation of tasks. It is logical to think that teaching students leadership concepts during their professional preparation would result in better leadership skills upon entering the workforce as clinicians and/or clinical supervisors. Benefits of incorporating peer leadership opportunities in the clinical education setting are summarized in Table 8-2.

IMPLEMENTING PEER LEADERSHIP

Peer leadership opportunities should be reserved for upperclassman or more experienced students due to the requisite clinical knowledge and maturity necessary for recognizing priorities in a hectic clinical environment. Your goals for implementing peer leadership should genuinely be educational in nature and not to alleviate your own workload by pawning off undesirable tasks in the clinical setting. Let us examine different ways you can incorporate leadership opportunities to benefit your students.

Athletic Trainer for the Day

One of the easiest approaches to implementing peer leadership is to make your upper level student the "athletic trainer for the day" (with your supervision of course). Inform the student the day before that he or she will be responsible for ensuring that all clinical duties are taken care of during the next session from pre-practice through post-practice. Without guidance, some students may become frustrated trying to multitask and prioritize the pre-practice needs of 10 patients (or more) at the same time while trying to ensure that field set-up occurs. More than likely, the student will attempt to accomplish most of the tasks alone and would never think to ask you to prepare coolers for practice! Allow the student to be the first person to evaluate any injuries that occur during practice that day and communicate decisions to the coaching staff. In addition, the peer leader would be responsible for ensuring all post-practice duties are completed.

Some of you may prefer the "sink or swim" approach to this exercise in which you provide little guidance on how to approach multitasking and planning and that allows the student to fail. Allowing the student to make mistakes (that do not harm patients) is not a bad approach because it requires reflective practice about what went well and what did not. In addition, you should encourage the student's peer(s) to provide feedback on his or her performance as a leader. To better prepare your student for this experience the second time around, have him or her list all of the activities that occur on a daily basis in the clinical setting and what time they typically occur. Next, the student should assign available personnel (peers and certified staff) to each task and communicate each person's responsibilities for the day. Emphasize to the student leader that unexpected events (ie, emergencies, weather, etc) can pop up at any time during the clinical session and they should be as proactive as possible in planning for such events by reviewing the emergency action plan ahead of time in order to appropriately delegate tasks in stressful situations.

This exercise can be a challenge for many ACIs because it requires a great deal of trust in the student's clinical knowledge. The key is to ensure that you are providing an adequate level of supervised autonomy and can step in on behalf of the patient should you feel that the student's decision will cause harm. This exercise can be applied in any clinical setting or situation such as game days, working with multiple patients in a rehabilitation clinic, or high school setting.

Student Rehabilitation Coordinator

One leadership opportunity that has been very successful is the development of a student rehabilitation coordinator for university settings with morning rehabilitation hours. In this environment, there are generally 3 to 4 hours in the morning set aside for all short- and long-term rehabilitation sessions for student-athletes, often resulting in 5 to 10 patients needing service at one time. Assigning a student leader in this environment is an excellent way to develop skills in multitasking and administration.

At the University of North Carolina at Greensboro, we assign all upper classman (eg, second year entry-level master's students) to 4 to 6 hours of morning rehabilitation per week with a student rehabilitation coordinator in this setting. The student rehabilitation coordinator serves as a peer leader and liaison with the athletic training staff (who provide constant supervision of all students). With a gradual decrease in guidance over time, the supervising ACI assists the peer leader in delegating tasks to his/her peers to ensure that all patients' needs are being met. In addition, the peer leader is responsible for ensuring that his/her peers are updating all patient files and the injury surveillance system on a daily basis. Because this experience also serves as a rehabilitation intensive experience for the peer leader, this student leader is also becoming more proficient in planning and implementing short- and long-term rehabilitation protocols. The peer leader is evaluated by an ACI, not only on rehabilitation skills, but on professional behaviors and leadership characteristics. This form of peer leadership is an excellent opportunity for those students who want to work in a collegiate athletic training setting with a high volume of patients. Likewise, this exercise in peer leadership could also be applied in an out-patient rehabilitation clinic that has more than one student assigned to an ACI who has a high patient load.

Special Events Coordinator

Another easy method of incorporating peer leadership opportunities is through the coordination of special events. It is very common for colleges/universities and high schools to host at least one major special event each year, whether it is a weekend volleyball tournament or a large conference track meet. As you know, such events often require extensive planning that goes beyond the typical game day coverage. While it may not be wise to turn over all of the planning of such events to upperclassman, they can be utilized to coordinate certain aspects of the event with your guidance. For example, students can easily write letters to visiting teams explaining what athletic training services and supplies will be available for their use, coordinate physician coverage, as well as set up a schedule for other students to volunteer for the event. They can also be in charge of event management tasks such as ensuring that the locker rooms and field/court are set up and restocked as needed with appropriate supplies. Offering these types of leadership opportunities provides students with a more realistic view of the real world duties of an athletic trainer that may not be fully captured in the classroom setting.

PEER MENTORING

Peer mentoring can be described as a supportive or nurturing relationship between two students of differing academic or experience levels within the professional program (eg, an upper level student mentoring a lower level student).[8,16] Peer mentoring focuses more on professional socialization,[15,23] emotional support, and encouragement rather than on peer teaching and learning.[15,23] Professional socialization is the process whereby individuals acquire the norms, values, knowledge, and skills that allow them to function in a particular role.[24]

Student perspectives on mentoring have been examined in the context of athletic training professional socialization.[25,26] While the majority of ATSs report that their mentor is a current practicing athletic trainer (eg, head athletic trainer), a small percentage indicate they viewed a peer as a mentor. This suggests that ATSs may assist in the professional socialization process.[25] In addition, ATSs identified the roles of mentors as being consistent with those reported in a nursing peer mentoring study (eg, emotional support, role modeling, giving advice).[25] As well, our previous research indicates that ATSs often seek advice from their peers while in the clinical setting.[4] Theoretically, these studies support the concept that ATSs could be potential mentors for their peers with multiple benefits for both the mentor and the protégé. Benefits of incorporating peer mentoring opportunities in the clinical education setting are summarized in Table 8-3.

TABLE 8-3

BENEFITS OF PEER MENTORING

BENEFITS FOR PEER MENTORS

- Increased sense of personal growth and development[23]
- Joy and satisfaction in helping others[23]
- Improved organizational skills[23,27]
- Enhanced self-reflection of own clinical practice and skills[23,27]
- Desire to mentor/teach students in the future[23,27]

BENEFITS FOR PEER "PROTÉGÉS"[23,27–29]

- Experienced less anxiety in the clinical setting
- Increased self-confidence
- Increased comfort in the clinical environment

INCORPORATING PEER MENTORING

Many students will certainly view you as their mentor. However, it is important to foster mentoring relationships among your students with the hopes that they will develop supportive attitudes for peers and students during their professional practice. Peer mentoring is not uncommon among ATEPs. In our experience, it is most effective for pre-athletic training students (pre-ATS) and underclassman. Think back to your days as an athletic training student. Many of you probably experienced some level of anxiety walking into the athletic training room for the first time and stood against the wall too afraid to ask any questions. Now, imagine if you had been paired with an upperclassman who was charged with "taking you under his/her wing" to orient you to the setting and serve as a role model. This type of prearranged mentoring relationship significantly reduces anxiety in the clinical setting.

Big Brother/Big Sister Model

One effective approach for incorporating peer mentoring with observation or pre-ATS is the big brother/big sister model. In this model, pre-ATSs are assigned to an upperclassman at the beginning of the semester with the purpose of orienting or socializing the younger student into the athletic training environment. This arrangement alleviates some role strain for the ACI. The peer mentor may be charged with initially meeting with the pre-ATS in a less formal environment to mutually share their interests in the field of athletic training. This may be followed with several hours of observing the peer mentor in the athletic training room and learning about the typical day of an ATS as well as a certified athletic trainer. It may be beneficial for the mentor to have a list of specific rudimentary tasks to complete with the pre-ATS. This could include touring the athletic facilities, locating specific supplies in the athletic training room, learning the names of all of the certified staff members, and practicing laboratory skills.

Lower-level students such as sophomores can also benefit from peer mentoring (from advanced students) as they are still beginning students in the ATEP. These students often have very basic foundational knowledge and skills and are not very efficient in completing tasks due to their lack of clinical experience. As a result, they may face challenges navigating the clinical environment and lack awareness or a sense of urgency regarding completing clinical tasks. Peer mentors can assist with socializing beginning students into the clinical setting by providing insight and advice on how to deal with certain situations. For example, a peer mentor will undoubtedly have more experience communicating with ACIs and therefore could coach beginning students on effective strategies for communicating with ACIs and others (eg, when it is appropriate to ask questions).

PEER ASSESSMENT/FEEDBACK

As students who teach their peers gain a deeper understanding of concepts, the same can be said when they assess or provide feedback to peers on their clinical performance. Peer assessment can be defined as students evaluating the products or outcomes of learning.[6] In the context of the clinical setting, this may include students providing one another with both formal and informal feedback about their clinical skill performance and professional behaviors and attitudes. As you can see, peer assessment/feedback can be used to "close the loop" on the other forms of PAL previously discussed.

Several benefits of peer assessment/feedback have been identified during allied health care professional preparation. Students will often take greater ownership in learning and retaining clinical knowledge and skills if they know they will be held accountable by their peers.[20] In addition, students gain valuable insight into the assessment process that may prove beneficial when they themselves are being evaluated, or when asked to conduct performance evaluations of employees in the future. Benefits of incorporating peer assessment/feedback opportunities in the clinical education setting are summarized in Table 8-4.

IMPLEMENTING PEER ASSESSMENT/FEEDBACK

Peer assessment/feedback can be implemented with a variety of goals in mind, such as improving performance of clinical skills, increasing the students' self-awareness of areas requiring improvement, and encouraging collaborative relationships in the clinical environment.[20] We will discuss several examples for incorporating this form of PAL in the clinical setting.

Many ATEPs utilize peer assessment/feedback in laboratory-based courses where research has shown students can accurately assess their peers' psychomotor skills.[34] This type of activity can also be useful in the clinical setting to fill "down time" between patients. Likewise, informal peer feedback can be just as useful in the clinical setting following patient interactions. For example, students can provide informal verbal feedback after observing one another during patient evaluations, rehabilitation sessions, or any other patient care situations. It is also useful to have peers formally evaluate one another's professional behaviors at the middle and end of a clinical rotation, similar to what you do as an ACI. This allows students to develop the ability to give and receive constructive feedback. Some research in other allied health disciplines[35] indi-

TABLE 8-4

Benefits of Peer Assessment/Feedback

- Gain insight into the assessment and feedback process[30]
- Gain experience in giving and receiving constructive criticism[31]
- Socializes students to seek constructive criticism and collegial interactions in future professional practice[31,32]
- Enhanced ability to self-identify areas for improvement[32,33]
- Greater insight into how they process information[20]
- Increased student motivation and ownership in the learning process[27]
- Increased retention of material[20]
- Enhanced self-esteem and self-respect[27]
- Improved cohesiveness between and within student cohorts[27]

cates that the feedback received from peers lacks sufficient detail compared to what you may provide. Therefore, it is important to use peer assessment/feedback only as a supplement to feedback from the ACI.

Summary

Various forms of PAL can be mutually beneficial for all students involved in the learning process. In addition, ACIs may lessen their role strain when implementing learning experiences that allow for educational exchanges between students.

Reflection Questions

Draw your own insights about how you can implement PAL in the clinical education setting by answering these questions:

- As the athletic trainer working with football, you are charged with providing adequate health care for 80 student-athletes. The director of the athletic training education program at your institution approaches you about becoming an ACI for the program. You are initially hesitant about adding the instruction and supervision of students to the laundry list of duties you complete on a daily basis. How can you implement PAL to assist you in successfully serving as an ACI without overloading your role as a health care provider?

- You have been assigned to supervise 3 athletic training students while working with the gymnastics team. One student is a sophomore, one is a junior, and the third is a senior. How can you foster optimal clinical education among these students with varying experience levels?

REFERENCES

1. Commission on Accreditation of Athletic Training Education. *Standards for the Accreditation of Entry Level Educational Programs for the Athletic Trainer.* Round Rock, TX: Author; 2006
2. Weidner TG, Henning JM. Importance and applicability of approved clinical instructor standards and criteria to certified athletic trainers in different clinical education settings. *J Athl Train.* 2005;40(4):326-332.
3. Henning JM, Weidner TG, Marty MC. Peer assisted learning in clinical education: literature review. *Athl Train Educ J* . 2008;3(Jul-Sep):84-90 .
4. Henning JM, Weidner TG, Jones J. Peer-assisted learning in the athletic training clinical setting. *J Athl Train.* 2006;41(1):102-108.
5. Vaidya SR. Improving teaching and learning through peer coaching. *Educ.* 1994;115(2):241-245.
6. Topping K, Ehly S, eds. *Peer-Assisted Learning.* Mahwah, NJ: Lawrence Erlbaum Associates; 1998.
7. Ammon K, Schroll NM. The junior student as peer leader. *Nursing Outlook.* 1988;36(2):85-86.
8. Weidner TG, Popp JK. Peer-assisted learning is effective in improving orthopedic evaluation psychomotor skills. *J Athl Train.* 2007;42(1): 113-119.
9. Rubin L, Hebert C. Model for active learning. *College Teaching.* 1998;46(1):26-30.
10. Lincoln MA, McAllister LL. Peer learning in clinical education. *Med Teach.* 1993;15(1):17-25.
11. Hendelman WJ. Reciprocal peer teaching by medical students in the gross anatomy laboratory. *J Med Educ.* 1986;61:674-680
12. Cason CL, Cason GJ, Bartnik DA. Peer instruction in professional nurse education: a qualitative case study. *J Nurs Educ.* 1977;16(7):10-22.
13. Glynn LG, MacFarlane A, Kelly M, Cantillon P, Murphy AW. Helping each other to learn: a process evaluation of peer-assisted learning. *BMC Med Educ.* 2006;6(18):1-9
14. Escovitz ES. Using senior students as clinical skills teaching assistants. *Acad Med.* 1990;65(12):733-734.
15. Aviram M, Ophir R, Raviv D, Shiloah M. Experiential learning of clinical skills by beginning nursing students: "coaching" project by fourth-year student interns. *J Nurs Educ.* 1998;37(5):228-231.
16. Iwasiw CL, Goldenberg D. Peer teaching among nursing students in the clinical area: effects on student learning. *J Adv Nurs.* 1993;18:659-668.
17. Bos S. Perceived benefits of peer leadership as described by junior baccalaureate nursing students. *J Nurs Educ.* 1998;37(4):189-191.
18. Emery MJ, Nalette E. Student-staffed clinics: creative clinical education during times of constraint. *Clin Manag Phys Ther.* 1986;6(2):6, 9-10.
19. Meyer LP. Athletic training clinical instructors as situational leaders. *J Athl Train.* 2002;37(4 Suppl): S261-S265.
20. Henning JM, Marty MC. A practical guide to implementing peer assessment in athletic training education. *Athletic Therapy Today.* 2008;13(3): 29-32
21. Burnside IM. Peer supervision: a method of teaching. *J Nurs Educ.* 1971;10(3):15-22.
22. Whitman NA. *Peer Teaching: To Teach Is to Learn Twice.* Washington, DC: Association for the Study of Higher Education; 1988.
23. Yates P, Cunningham J, Moyle W, Wollin J. Peer mentorship in clinical education: outcomes of a pilot programme for first year students. *Nurse Educ Today.* 1997;17:508-514.
24. McPherson BD. Socialization into and through sport involvement. In: Luschen GRF, Sage GH, eds. *Handbook of Social Science of Sport.* Champaign, IL: Stipes; 1981:246-273.
25. Pitney WA, Ehlers G, Walker S. A descriptive study of athletic training students' perceptions of effective mentoring roles. *IJAHSP.* 2006;4(2):1-8.
26. Pitney WA, Ehlers G. A grounded theory study of the mentoring process involved with undergraduate athletic training students. *J Athl Train.* 2004;39(4):344-351.
27. Costello J. Learning from each other: peer teaching and learning in student nurse training. *Nurse Educ Today.* 1989;9:203-206.
28. Scott ES. Peer-to-peer mentoring: teaching collegiality. *Nurse Educ.* 2005;30(2):52-56.
29. Glass N, Walter R. An experience of peer mentoring with student nurses: enhancement of personal and professional growth. *J Nurs Educ.* 2000;39(4):155-160.
30. Topping K. Peer assessment between students in colleges and universities. *Rev Educ Res.* 1998;68(3):249-276.
31. Gerace L, Sibilano H. Preparing students for peer collaboration: a clinical teaching model. *J Nurs Educ.* 2006;23(5):206-209.
32. Erickson GP. Peer evaluation as a teaching-learning strategy in baccalaureate education for community health nursing. *J Nurs Educ.* 1987;26(5):204-206.

33. Flynn JP, Marcus MT, Schmadl JC. Peer review: a successful teaching strategy in baccalaureate education. *J Nurs Educ.* 1981;23(5):28-32.
34. Marty MC, Henning JM, Willse JT. Students are reliable assessing a peer performing an athletic training psychomotor skill. *J Athl Train.* 2008;43(3 Suppl):S-90.
35. Ladyshewsky R, Gotjamanos E. Communication skill development in health professional education: the use of standardized patients in combination with a peer assessment strategy. *J Allied Health.* 1997; 26(4):177-186

The Supervision, Questioning, Feedback Model of Clinical Teaching
A Practical Approach

Mary G. Barnum, EdD, ATC, LAT; M. Susan Guyer, DPE, ATC, LAT, CSCS;
Linda S. Levy, EdD, ATC; and Carrie Graham, MA, ATC, LAT

Approved clinical instructors (ACIs) are busy people who have multiple responsibilities. You are a health care provider, an administrator, and an educator, to name just a few. With so much information about educational theories and teaching tools, it can be difficult and overwhelming to know where to start. We hope to provide you with an easy-to-understand and easy-to-use model of clinical teaching, the Supervision, Questioning, Feedback (SQF) Model. The SQF model of clinical teaching, depicted in Figure 9-1, practically integrates **S**upervision, **Q**uestioning, and **F**eedback into the clinical learning experiences that you provide for your students. The SQF model is grounded in the concept that clinical learning is experiential, and that clinical teaching requires a different approach than does teaching in the traditional classroom setting. When examining experiential learning models, 3 dimensions are constant: 1) the instructor serves as a facilitator and supervisor of learning, coming in and out of the learning experience as needed to assist the student in reaching the outcomes identified for that specific experience; 2) instructors ask questions throughout the learning experience for the expressed purpose of stimulating the student to think or process information in a specific way or for a specific outcome; and 3) feedback is given at different times, in different ways, for different reasons. As the student's knowledge and skills develop and expand through clinical experiences, the way in which the ACI uses supervision, questioning, and feedback will be modified. The purpose of this chapter is to describe and explain how each element of the SQF Model of Clinical Teaching, as depicted in Figure 9-1, works and to demonstrate how each element fits together to provide an interactive model for clinical teaching.

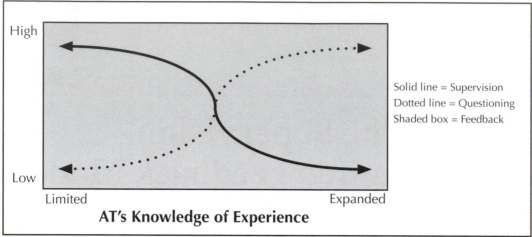

Figure 9-1. SQF Model of Clinical Teaching—supervision, questioning, and feedback components. For students whose knowledge and experience is limited, situational supervision is high, meaning the ACI very closely monitors the student's actions, providing constant direction. As the student's knowledge and experience base begins expanding, situational supervision begins to be less intense or lower, meaning that the approved clinical instructor gradually begins to allow greater student autonomy in decision making while still monitoring student's actions. In contrast, the level of questioning transition is the opposite, with students needing more low-level questions initially, when knowledge and experiences are limited. As experience and knowledge expand, students need to be asked more high-level questions. Feedback is provided constantly throughout all interactions with students.

SUPERVISION: THE "S" IN SQF

Supervision implies a watching over and suggests a passive involvement. However, clinical teaching requires that you as the ACI be actively involved. The supervision that you provide should be dependent upon the learning that needs to take place. We call this type of supervision situational. Situational supervision is dynamic, active, and interactive, combining aspects of both teaching and supervising.

Situational supervision is based on the premise that supervision should take into account the needs of the student based on his or her developmental level (ie, knowledge, skills, and experiences).[1,2] Novice athletic training students (ATSs) have minimal knowledge and skills, while advanced ATSs who are nearing the completion of their studies have expanded knowledge and skills. The underlying premise of situational supervision is that the ACI should utilize a supervisory style that matches the ATSs developmental level and that supports student growth and competence.[2,3]

STUDENT DEVELOPMENT LEVELS AND ACI SUPERVISION

Student developmental levels within the situational supervision model are divided into 4 quadrants: D1/D2) novice learner, D3) intermediate learner, and D4) autonomous learner.[4] ACI supervision behaviors correspond with the ATSs developmental level and are termed as S1/S2) directing and coaching, S3) supporting, and S4) delegating.[4] Characteristics associated with the ATSs' development level and your corresponding supervision behaviors can be found in Table 9-1. For students who have limited knowledge and experiences, the situational supervision is high, constant and close, consisting of directing and coaching. As the student's knowledge and experience base begins to expand, supervision transitions to moderate, constant, and more distant and consists of coaching and supporting. With students who have a more vast knowledge and experience base, the supervision style, consisting of supporting and delegating, is low, yet constant, allowing greater autonomy.[4-6]

Although the situational supervision model appears sequential and orderly, learning is a highly complex phenomenon. An ATS typically begins his or her journey stages as a *novice learner* and progresses into the *autonomous learner*. The following narratives are examples of how the situational supervision model works. With each example, we have indicated the following: 1) ACI supervision behavior; 2) student's developmental level; and 3) information present within the scenario that helps the ACI determine which supervision behavior is needed. Some information is present within the scenario, while other information is not and should be gathered prior to the student beginning his or her clinical rotation. This information is generally obtained from various sources such as the course syllabi and evaluations/remarks from previous ACIs who have worked with a particular student.

EXAMPLE 1

In Emily's injury assessment class this week, she learned and practiced all of the tests that need to be completed following a suspected ankle sprain. That afternoon, during her first clinical assignment with the men's basketball team, a player came down from a rebound inverting his ankle. Emily was so eager to try out her new skills that her ACI allowed her to conduct the injury assessment. With her ACI kneeling beside her and watching intently, Emily began by collecting the appropriate pertinent information through the history taking process and then quickly moved to palpating as many structures as she could remember.

As she began the range of motion testing, as she had been taught in her assessment course, her actions caused her patient pain. She then attempted an inversion stress test but had difficulty securing the joint because of the athlete's footwear. At this point, the ACI tells Emily, "OK, let's stop there. Watch me and I want you to compare what you did with what I am doing." Emily was surprised at how different her ACI's evaluation was compared to her own. The feedback Emily received reminded her that she had more to learn and practice before she attempted to assess another injury. The next time she attempted to perform an ankle evaluation, Emily turned to her ACI after each section of her evaluation and looked for approval that she was doing everything correctly and in the proper order. Her ACI provided clear directions for Emily and stated, "Your history is complete and you have palpated all the appropriate structures; now begin your range of motion testing."

Information:
ACI Supervision Behavior:　　　　S1/S2—Directing and coaching
Student Developmental Level:　　　D1/D2—Novice Learner

Information used to determine student developmental level:
- Based on student's academic level in program and observations of student during the clinical experience, the student is determined to have limited knowledge and skill.
- First clinical rotation with no "real-life" experiences from which to draw.

TABLE 9-1

ATHLETIC TRAINING STUDENT DEVELOPMENTAL CHARACTERISTICS

DEVELOPMENTAL LEVEL	LEARNER CHARACTERISTICS	APPROVED CLINICAL INSTRUCTOR SITUATIONAL SUPERVISION BEHAVIORS	QUESTIONING LEVEL	FEEDBACK
D1→ Novice learner: eager novice	Enthusiastic and eager to perform newly acquired athletic training knowledge from the classroom in the laboratory settings. Confident in his or her skills and knowledge yet really does not comprehend the complexity of the information nor truly possesses the ability to apply it in real-life situations. When asked to perform skills in the clinical setting, the eager novice may stumble through the task because it is not yet practiced.	S1→ Directing and motivation Provides clear directions and corrective feedback. Provides close and consistent contact with the student. Checks for understanding of task. Instructs on how to complete the task successfully.	Most of the questions that will be asked will be at the "what" level in order to check student's knowledge base and confirm accuracy of response. Some questions should be asked at the "so what" level with minimal questions asked at the "now what" level.	Utilize primarily corrective feedback.
D2→ Novice learner: early competence	Gained an awareness that his or her body of knowledge and skill base is quite limited compared to what is needed to successfully function independently as an athletic trainer. The student may realize that his or her depth of understanding was less than first anticipated or is not able to complete the task as completely or well as expected. Self-confidence may be lower than the ATS in the D1 stage of development. Not able to perform tasks satisfactorily	S2→ Coaching and motivating Provides directive feedback, cues, and tips for completing a task as well as affirming and supportive statements that allow the student to work through the challenge. ATS is still learning the task and may be feeling frustrated if the task was more difficult than had been anticipated. Feedback is sincere, specific, and timely to reinforce the desired outcome of the skill or interaction.	Most of the questions that will be asked will be at the "what" level in order to check student's knowledge base and confirm accuracy of response. Some questions should be asked at the "so what" level with minimal questions asked at the "now what" level.	Utilize primarily corrective feedback transitioning to directive feedback when student demonstrates competence in an area.

continued

TABLE 9-1 continued

ATHLETIC TRAINING STUDENT DEVELOPMENTAL CHARACTERISTICS

DEVELOPMENTAL LEVEL	LEARNER CHARACTERISTICS	APPROVED CLINICAL INSTRUCTOR SITUATIONAL SUPERVISION BEHAVIORS	QUESTIONING LEVEL	FEEDBACK
D3→ *Intermediate learner: situationally proficient learner*	Is becoming more proficient and competent at performing skills as they are practiced and improved during clinical learning experiences. Takes longer to make decisions and perform skills as earlier self-doubt is slowly replaced with confidence in decision-making and skill application abilities. Gaining confidence yet is still cautious about his or her abilities.	**S3→ Supporting and motivating** Involves allowing the student to problem solve and discover solutions without stepping in and giving immediate solutions. Provides the student clear, specific encouragement and recognition for the achievement of the desired task.	Begin interaction with "what" level questions, but quickly transition to "so what" level questions, asking primarily "so what" level questions with a few "now what" questions.	Provide equal amounts of corrective and directive feedback.
D4→ *Autonomous learner*	Has the knowledge, confidence, and competence to complete the necessary athletic training skills in the clinical setting as ability to utilize his or her knowledge and skill base becomes more efficient.6 Actively engages patients to provide assessment and treatment services and embraces opportunities that assist them in expanding and refining their knowledge and skill base	**S4→ Delegating and motivating** Provides reflective feedback, greater autonomy, challenging knowledge and skill base through higher level strategic questioning and affirmation of well conceived and executed patient interactions. Needs very little, if any, direction and support. Demonstrates competence and commitment to the task and has become self-managed.	Majority of questions will be posed at the "now what" level but will need to utilize "what" and "so what" to build platform for "now what" questions.	Provide mostly directive feedback using corrective only as needed.

- Has false sense of abilities (eager to attempt an on-field acute evaluation with no experience in doing so).

- Starts strong but does not know how to respond appropriately when faced with "real" patient reactions.

- In subsequent interactions, student demonstrates greater awareness of own limitations, seeks out guidance from ACI, and is able to utilize previous experiences to inform current situations.

EXAMPLE 2

Emily was in her second clinical rotation and completed the lower extremity orthopedic assessment course. In this current scenario, Emily had assessed an athlete's knee injury on the sidelines during practice. Feeling more confident about her injury assessment skills, Emily has moved into the intermediate learner stage and has independently assumed the challenge of determining the nature and severity of this athlete's complaints.

Her ACI stood close enough to watch and hear the interactions but allowed the interaction between Emily and the patient to take place naturally. Emily completed her evaluation in proper sequence but did not perform individual manual muscle testing for each muscle within the hamstring group. Her ACI also noticed that she was having trouble with the Lachman's ACL test. At the conclusion of her evaluation, she turned to her ACI for feedback. The ACI made statements such as, "Emily, the evaluation you are completing is clearly ruling out some possible causes of this patient's pain. However, I am wondering if we should look more closely together at the individual hamstrings, and maybe try some alternative ACL test to make sure we didn't miss anything. What are your thoughts?" These supportive questions prompted Emily to reflect on the way she had assessed both the hamstrings and ACL and prompted her to perform additional testing.

Information:
ACI Supervision Behavior: S3—Supporting
Student Developmental Level: D3—Intermediate Learner

Information used to determine student developmental level:
- Since Emily has completed the lower extremity orthopedic assessment course, assumption is made that she has the basic knowledge and skills to assess the athlete's injury. Also, since she is currently in her second rotation, she has developed some confidence and awareness of how to complete an evaluation with a real patient. Scores from her first rotation, as well as remarks from her first ACI, indicate she is a strong student for her grade level and experience.

- Emily appears confident and completes her evaluation with only minor mistakes.

- Emily does not look to her ACI for confirmation or assistance during the process but does seek feedback at the conclusion of the evaluation.

EXAMPLE 3

Now in her third clinical experience, Emily once again had to assess an injury. This time, an athlete came into the athletic training room complaining of shoulder pain from baseball pitching. Emily was given permission to complete the assessment. With her ACI watching, Emily was able to complete the assessment from beginning to end without ACI intervention. She demonstrated confidence in her knowledge and abilities by the way she interacted with the patient, moved through her evaluation, and arrived at the diagnosis. At this point, the ACI provided positive and affirming feedback and posed such questions as, "Identify for me all the components of your evaluation that support your diagnosis," "Explain to me how you ruled out conditions that present similar to this one," or "I agree with your diagnosis, tell me how we should proceed with treating this patient." Additional feedback was provided that encouraged her continued advancement toward autonomy.

Information:
ACI Supervision Behavior: S4—Delegating
Student Developmental Level: D4—Autonomous learner

Information used to determine student developmental level:

- Based on Emily's academic level in program, review of previous coursework, and evaluations, she is determined to have developed an advanced skill and knowledge base.

- Emily's skill application has become second nature; she can perform skills and answer questions at same time, demonstrating confidence in abilities.

- Emily seeks ACI permission to evaluate but does not need additional information or direction from the ACI in order to complete the evaluation. She confidently and accurately shares her findings with the ACI and indicates correct treatment plan.

Even though these scenarios are fictitious, Emily's struggles at the beginning of her clinical experiences certainly mimic first-year clinical students. Emily's ACI was able to provide her with the type of feedback that prevented her from giving up or from thinking that everything she did was fine and that she did not need to be supervised. Emily's development as an ATS move her from the novice learner to the autonomous learner, with supervision that encouraged confidence building and skill proficiency.[4-6]

QUESTIONING: THE "Q" IN SQF

As an ACI, you need to ask your students questions. Asking questions serves several different purposes. Some questions are posed in order to "check" the student's knowledge base and verify that he or she accurately comprehends that knowledge.[7] Some questions require the student to respond by applying his or her knowledge either by word or action. Questions can also be used to stimulate critical thinking.[8] One of the key concepts when utilizing questioning strategically is that each question needs to be phrased in a certain way in order to stimulate a different thought process.[9-11] Let us look at the different types of questions that you can ask in order to make a student think in different ways about the content he or she is learning.

TABLE 9-2

LEVELS OF QUESTIONING, CHARACTERISTICS, AND EXAMPLES

STRATEGIC QUESTIONING

Level of Questioning	Characteristics	Examples
What	Targets lower-level processing skills, declarative knowledge, application, and comprehension.	Identify the sequence in which… Which stage of healing…? What is the primary…? Explain to me… Who are the…?
So What	Intended to move the student from using lower-level thinking processes to higher, more complex ways of thinking about the information. Requires the student to utilize stored knowledge. Compares current knowledge with what he or she is seeing, hearing, and doing.	Compare information from…? Summarize for me the…? How is this different from…? What other options should we consider?
Now What	Questions require the student to evaluate the information and determine appropriate responses or plans; infer meaning, project outcomes, defend his or her decisions, or challenge assumptions. Target the thinking processes vital for developing the ability to critically consider information and in developing clinical reasoning skills.	Tell me what you believe … How did you come to your conclusion? What do you think…? If X happens, how will Y be affected?

QUESTIONING LEVELS

Borrowing from experiential learning research,[10] questions can be categorized into 3 levels: what, so what, and now what (Table 9-2). When posing any question, it is recommended that you allow 3 to 5 seconds for the students to process the question before they respond to the question.[12]

"WHAT" LEVEL QUESTIONS

"What" level questions target the least complex type of thinking, and are associated with declarative knowledge, application, and comprehension.[9,10] When you ask a student questions at the "what" level, you are asking him or her to list, describe, define, point out, identify, apply, use, or select. With these questions, you are making the student look at a given situation and identify just the basics or facts of what he or she knows to be true.[9,10] For example, can they correctly identify the padding material being used? Can they accurately describe the principle governing how a specific material used in protective padding interacts with a given force?

"What" level questions are the initial starting point when using strategic questioning with students, meaning that all students, regardless of their developmental level, should be asked "what" level questions first. However, how many "what" level questions you ask and the complexity of the content targeted by the question will differ based upon the student's knowledge, skills, and experiences. "What" level questions are used to confirm for both the student and the ACI that the student's knowledge and understanding of a concept is accurate or that the student can correctly apply information or perform a skill. In the 3 examples presented below, we will follow a student through a scenario to see how to phrase questions using the "what, so-what, now-what" sequence. This first example demonstrates how to utilize "what" level questions during your students' clinical learning experiences. The purpose in asking these specific questions is to stimulate the student to recall information acquired in previous courses and experiences, check the student's comprehension of the information acquired in previous courses and experiences, and build a platform of knowledge from which more complex information and questions will be generated.[9] Also notice that not all questions contain the word *what*. Because the goal is to stimulate thinking that is associated with knowledge (what do they know), comprehension (what do they understand), and application (how they apply their knowledge),[9-11] "what" level questions can include words such as *how*, *show*, *describe*, and *explain*.

Scenario

Your institution is hosting the Regional Cross-Country Championships and you are in the beginning stages of organizing athletic health care services for this event. You decide to include your sophomore student in the planning process. The student has completed an injury prevention and risk management course the previous semester but has not yet had an administration course. This is the student's first clinical rotation. You begin your discussion with the student by asking him a series of "what" level questions:

- "Where would you go to determine the type of injuries that typically occur during elite cross country running events?"
- "How should we go about determining how many athletes are expected to participate in this event?"
- "What are the primary types of supplies that we need to have on site?"
- "Explain to me our procedure for activating EMS."

There is no specific number of "what" level questions that could be asked. Once you have completed questioning at this level, it is time to move to the "so what" level.

"SO WHAT" LEVEL QUESTIONS

"So what" questions are intended to move the student from using lower-level thinking to higher, more complex ways of thinking about the information he or she is learning during his or her clinical experiences.[9,10] "So what" questions require the student to utilize stored knowledge or things that he or she already "knows" and compare that information with what he or she is seeing, hearing, and doing in the clinical setting.[9-11] At this level, you are asking the student to compare, synthesize, and analyze information.[9,11] We will build upon the example described previously to demonstrate the difference between "what" and "so what" level questions. Because the goal is to stimulate thinking needed to compare, synthesize, and analyze information, "so what" level questions may include terms such as *compare*, *pull together*, *integrate*, *examine*, *question*, or *analyze*.

You have completed asking the student several questions at the "what" level and are ready to ask questions at the "so what" level. The purpose in asking questions at the "so what" level is to assist the student in sorting through and organizing the information he or she is collecting, comparing information presented in the current scenario (or real life) with his or her textbook knowledge, and pulling together information from a variety of sources for analysis.

Scenario

- "How does the number of athletic trainers that we have determined are needed for this event compare with the NCAA recommendations"?

- "How does the process we used for determining the number of supplies needed for this event compare with the process outlined in your textbook"?

- "When you look at the *NCAA Sports Medicine Handbook*, our own policies, and the information in the textbook, what are the major common points that are seen among all of these sources"?

As with "what" level questions, there is no specific number of "so what" level questions that must be asked. That will depend upon the student's responses. Also, remember that the complexity of the content targeted within the question must be appropriate for the student's knowledge, skill, and experience. The third and final level of questioning is "now what."

"NOW WHAT" LEVEL QUESTIONS

"Now what"[10] questions require the student to evaluate the information and determine appropriate responses or plans, infer meaning, speculate on what might happen based on his or her actions or decisions, defend his or her decisions, or challenge his or her assumptions.[9-11,13] "Now what" questions target thinking vital for developing the ability to critically consider information and developing clinical reasoning skills.[9,14] "Now what" questions should target topics for which the student has strong knowledge and experience and should be directed at students who are both confident and competent.[5,9] For students who are less confident and/or have less knowledge and experience, the "now what" level questions need to be less demanding than those asked of the more advanced student. In other words, you need to make the questions difficult enough to stimulate active processing of the information and advance the student's knowledge, skills, and critical thinking without frustrating, defeating, or embarrassing the student. We will return to the same example regarding providing coverage for the cross-country championship to demonstrate "now what" level questions.

Scenario

Continuation of discussion with the sophomore student in which you are now ready to ask the student "what now" level questions.

- "Tell me what you believe our top 3 priorities should be for this event and why you have selected each."

- "If 2 different members of the planning team give you different opinions on how to prepare for this event, how do you go about determining whose advice to follow? How did you come to your conclusion?"

- "What do you think might be some of the challenges or obstacles that we might face in implementing our plan?"

The number of questions you pose at the "now level" and the complexity of content that is targeted are determined by the student's responses. Because you are asking questions that require the student to use critical thinking skills, "now what" questions are the most challenging for the student to process; and he or she will likely need a little more time in which to respond. When posing "now what" questions, include terms such as *determine*, *assess*, or *defend*, or phrases such as *state your opinion*. Allow the student to tell you how and why he or she has chosen a specific course of action or come to a specific conclusion.

The example provided in the scenario focused on a young, less experienced sophomore student. However, all levels of questioning are used with all students. It the difficulty of content as well as the number of questions asked at each level that should be adapted to match the developmental level of the student whom the ACI is engaging. As depicted in Figure 9-1, for students like the one in the example who have limited knowledge and skill, the majority of questions posed should be at the "what" and "so what" levels, with only one to two "now what" questions in each strategic questioning session. The opposite holds true for students with advanced knowledge, skill, and experience. You begin the interaction with a few "what" questions, but the majority of questions should be at the "so what" and "now what" levels. "What" and "so what" questions reinforce and build upon the student's knowledge acquired in the classroom and clinical experiences.[9] "Now what" questions challenge and expand. You need to listen to not only the accuracy of the response, but the confidence with which the student responds to help you determine when it is appropriate to ask more difficult and challenging questions and switch to the next questioning level.

STRATEGIC QUESTIONING

Strategic questioning involves asking questions that first establish the student's current level of knowledge and skill, reinforce basic or foundational knowledge, and then gradually transition the student from processing information using lower-level thinking skills to using higher-level thinking skills. We refer to this as strategic questioning. It involves using a plan or strategy to move the student through the different levels of thinking about information. Strategic questioners utilize, "what," "so what," and "now what"[10] questions repeatedly so that students begin to anticipate what type of question will be posed next. In doing so, the students learn how to think and not just what to think.[9] Students need to develop critical thinking and clinical reasoning skills in addition to technical expertise.[7-15] As an ACI, strategic questioning is an important skill for you to acquire.

COMBINING SUPERVISION AND QUESTIONING

When comparing the level of supervision provided with the type of questions you should be asking (see Figure 9-1), note that while inexperienced novice students (students at the D1/D2 development levels) need high levels of supervision and lots of coaching and directing, they need to be asked low-level questions. This makes sense because less experienced and less knowledgeable students are often apprehensive and unsure and look to you for confirmation that what they are doing, thinking, and saying are correct. Therefore, the ACI supervision behavior is close and frequent and consists of directing and coaching the students. Check the student's knowledge, skills, and level of understanding through using "what" level questions to confirm for both yourself and the student that he or she is on the right track. As student confidence and competence expands into the intermediate learner stage (D3), the ACI supervision behavior changes to supportive. This enables the student to perceive that he or she is moving toward autonomy (even though you are still keeping "tabs" on him or her). Now is the time to ask "so what" level questions, which are considered higher-level questions. Finally, the autonomous learner (students at the D4 development level) needs you to delegate and perhaps supervise from a greater distance, allowing that student to develop greater autonomy. At this point, it is vital that you are using questions that stimulate higher-order thinking about information, enabling the student to develop into a skilled critical thinker.

FEEDBACK: THE "F" IN SQF

Athletic training education is grounded in clinical skill "competency" and "proficiency."[16] Clinical skill competency suggests that athletic training students are able to correctly perform a specific clinical skill (eg, the student can demonstrate a Lachman's special test). This would include proper hand placement, direction of force, etc, which would elicit accurate findings regarding cruciate laxity. Proficiency suggests the student has an ability to perform a skill correctly across a variety of circumstances and accurately interpret the findings. For example, can the same student who correctly performed the Lachman's test in a laboratory setting (and is therefore competent) appropriately utilize the test in the clinical setting with regard to selecting, assessing results, and recording findings? If so, that student is deemed proficient at performing and assessing findings for the Lachman's test. In your efforts to foster the student's competency and proficiency development, he or she will need appropriate feedback.

Feedback is the instruction, direction, comments, and examples you provide to the student regarding the student's application of his or her knowledge and skills.[17] Feedback should be specific, timely, clearly articulated and related to the outcomes identified for the specific task the student is attempting to complete. How the ACI delivers the feedback is also important. Students value ACIs that have good communication and instructional skills, optimize learning opportunities, provide clear and immediate feedback,[18] and demonstrate sensitivity to student needs.[19] We divide feedback into 2 types: corrective and directive.

Corrective Feedback

Corrective feedback lets the student know if his or her knowledge and skills are correctly being applied. Simply put, is what the student states accurate, and is he or she applying his or her skills correctly? Corrective feedback works on developing a student's basic knowledge and skills. It is used more often with novice students. As it is important not to let students develop incorrect techniques or believe inaccurate statements, corrective feedback needs to be used often. Corrective statements should be provided in a non-confrontational way and, if at all possible, not in front of patients or peers.

Directive Feedback

Directive feedback guides the student toward seeing different possibilities to rethink how he or she performed a specific task or responded to a question. Directive feedback can also involve guiding the student toward using additional resources to improve the quality of his or her response or action. Directive feedback is used when the student has the concept, skill, or information essentially correct, but perhaps certain aspects need refining, clarifying, or improving. As such, directive feedback will be used more often with advanced students. While corrective feedback lets the student know what he or she did wrong and how to correct it, directive feedback actively engages the student in considering different parts of his or her response or action in determining how to do it better or more efficiently. Whether feedback is being provided via corrective or directive statements, it is important to be clear and specific so that it relates action to outcome. If not, it can become a guessing game for the student, especially when there are multiple ways to achieve similar outcomes, yet the ACI is looking for only one, very specific answer. In the scenarios that follow, we will provide you examples of both corrective and directive feedback for the same student behavior.

Scenario 1

Student: "My patient's blister looks infected. I am going to scrub it out with peroxide, okay?

ACI corrective feedback statement: "You are correct. This site is infected; however, peroxide is not the appropriate solution to use in this situation. Let's debride the site using high pressure sterile saline and see what we have."

- In this example, the instructor has confirmed the student's assessment, indicated that his or her choice of treatment is incorrect, and told him or her which treatment option to utilize. Best used for novice learners in the D1 and D2 development level.

ACI directive feedback statement: "I agree it looks infected. Peroxide is a very harsh treatment. What other options are available to you to treat this condition?"

- In this example, the instructor has also confirmed the student's assessment, indicated that the student's choice of treatment is incorrect, but has now directed the student to consider other options that will require the student to seek out new information in order to proceed. Appropriate for autonomous learners in the D3 and D4 development levels.

Scenario 2

Student: "I got a positive apprehension test, so I think this patient has a dislocated patella."

Corrective feedback statement: "You performed the test correctly, and I agree the test was positive. However, considering the history, no obvious deformity, and a positive apprehension test, you have confirmed the presence of a patellar subluxation, not dislocation."

- In this example, the instructor has confirmed that the student's skill application and choice of tests were correct but that his or her assessment of the findings is incorrect. The instructor has provided the correct interpretation for the student and the feedback is very specific. Most appropriate for novice students D1 and D2 developmental levels.

Directive feedback statement: "You performed the test correctly, and I agree that the response was positive. Your final assessment is close, but I believe you may have overlooked key findings in the history and inspection phase of your evaluation to support a diagnosis of dislocation. Take a moment to analyze your findings in order to reconsider your final assessment."

- Again, the instructor confirms for the student what was done correctly, yet alerts the student to some weaknesses within the evaluation process. However, instead of providing the answer for the student, the instructor directs the student to reconsider the specific parts of the evaluation where important information was missed. Most appropriate for autonomous students at the D4 developmental level.

As represented in Figure 9-1 (gray background), feedback is constantly provided to your students. It should be given on a daily basis during clinical experiences. The feedback needs to be constructive in order to achieve a specific outcome within a specific situation. Corrective feedback is more appropriate to use with novice learners, especially in situations in which you will need to intervene to avoid injurious consequences. Directive feedback is more appropriate to use with developing intermediate and autonomous learners whose skill, knowledge, and experience base is expanding. As with supervision and questioning, the type of feedback you provide is dependent upon the abilities and needs of the learner.

CONCLUSION

In the SQF Model of Clinical Teaching, clinical teaching begins and ends with the learner. The key to using this model is to first appropriately recognize the student's developmental level. Once you become adept at determining whether a student is a novice, intermediate, or autonomous learner, you then match up supervision strategic questioning and feedback levels in order to move the student from being totally dependent on you for correct skill application and decision making to becoming a clinically proficient critical thinker. In general, novice learners need to be directed and coached, asked mainly "what" level questions, and given corrective feedback. Intermediate learners need to be supported, asked mainly "so what" level questions, and given a combination of corrective and directive feedback. For autonomous learners, primarily use a delegating style of supervision, ask mainly "now what" level questions, and provide directive feedback.

REFLECTION QUESTIONS

- What type of supervision behaviors do you exhibit most often?
- Think of several different interactions you have had with students and identify which of the following supervision behaviors would be most appropriate to use in each situation: directing, coaching, supporting, and delegating.
- What level of questions do you use most often?

- Practice your strategic questioning skills by thinking of a typical interaction you might have with a student and then plan out a sequence of questions that uses the "what," "so what," and "now what" levels of questioning.

- How would you describe the type of feedback that you typically provide to your students?

- Describe interactions with your students in which using corrective feedback would be the most appropriate type to provide. Directive feedback?

- How can you improve the clinical education experiences of your students based on the SQF model?

REFERENCES

1. Blanchard K, Hersey P. Great ideas revisited. *Training & Development.* 1996;(50)1:42-48.
2. Gates P, Blanchard K, Hersey P. Diagnosing educational leadership problems: a situational approach. *Educational Leadership.* 1976;33(5):348-354.
3. Hambleton R. Gumbert R. The validity of Hersey and Blanchard's theory of leader effectiveness. *Group & Organizational Studies.* 1982;7(2):225-242.
4. Blanchard K. Recognition and situational leadership II. *Emergency Librarian.* 1997;24(4):38.
5. Blanchard K, Nelson B. Where do you fit in? *Incentive.* 1996;170(10):65-66.
6. Guyer MS. *Factors That Influence Athletic Training Students' Cognition and Problem Solving Abilities.* Springfield, MA: Springfield College: 2003.
7. Cunningham RT. What kind of question is that? In: Wilen WW, ed. *Questioning Techniques and Effective Teaching.* Washington, DC: National Education Association; 1987:67-94.
8. King A. Designing the instructional process to enhance critical thinking across the curriculum: inquiring minds really do want to know: using questioning to teaching critical thinking. *Teach Psyc.* 1995;22:13-17.
9. Barnum M. Questioning skills demonstrated by approved clinical instructors during clinical field experiences. *J Athl Train.* 2008;43:284-292.
10. Priest S, Gass M. *Effective Leadership in Adventure Programming.* Champaign, IL: Human Kinetics; 1997.
11. Bloom BS. *Taxonomy of Educational Objectives Handbook One: Cognitive Domain.* London: Longmans; 1956.
12. Rowe MB. Wait time: slowing down may be a way of speeding up. *J Teach Educ.* 1986:43-49.
13. Orlich DC, Harder RJ, Callahan RC, et al. Deciding how to ask questions. *Teaching Strategies: A Guide to Better Instruction.* Lexington, MA: DC Health and Company; 1990:P187-226.
14. Phillips N, Duke M. The questioning skills of clinical teachers and preceptors: a comparative study. *J Adv Nur.* 2001;33:523-529.
15. Benner P. From novice to expert. *Am J Nur.* 1982;82:402-407.
16. Barnum MG, Guyer MS. Questioning and feedback in clinical education. *Athl Train Educ J.* In press.
17. Barnum MG, Graham C. Providing feedback to students on written assignments. *Athl Ther Today.* 2008; (13)5:2-5.
18. Weidner TG, Laurent T. Clinical instructors' and student athletic trainer perceptions of helpful clinical instructor characteristics. *J Athl Train.* 2001;36(1):58-61.
19. Jarski RW, Kulig K, Olson RE. Clinical teaching in physical therapy: student and teacher perceptions. *Phys Ther.* 1990;70:173-178.

The One-Minute Preceptor
A Time Efficient Clinical Teaching Model

Jolene M. Henning, EdD, ATC, LAT

It is well known that athletic training ACIs experience role strain while balancing patient care and clinical teaching in a busy athletic training room.[1] You have probably experienced strain in trying to figure out how to incorporate students into the patient care equation without affecting your productivity. ACIs would benefit from a clinical teaching model that addresses this delicate balance. Clinical teachers in medicine and nursing have mastered the One-Minute Preceptor (OMP) model of clinical teaching that is both time efficient and effective for teaching students in high-volume outpatient clinical settings. Clinical instructors trained in the OMP report being able to very quickly "diagnose" a student's knowledge and gain insight into his or her thought process.[2] In addition, they report being able to provide students with more specific and meaningful feedback regarding their clinical skills and knowledge. While a typical clinical teaching encounter takes longer than 1 minute, the essence is that the exchange is focused and brief. This chapter will help you to identify the 5 micro skills of the OMP model of clinical teaching, explain how each skill fosters effective teaching and facilitates student learning, and apply the skills of the OMP to patient scenarios.

THE FIVE MICRO-SKILLS

The OMP is a learner-centered approach to clinical teaching. It was introduced by clinical teachers (ie, preceptors) in medicine.[2] The OMP model can be used to guide any clinical teaching exchange and is composed of 5 micro-skills (Table 10-1) that we will briefly explore.

GET A COMMITMENT

The first step in the OMP involves getting a commitment from the student about what he or she thinks is wrong with the patient. The objective is to get the student to process and communicate information he or she has obtained from the patient.

TABLE 10-1

FIVE MICROSKILLS OF THE ONE-MINUTE PRECEPTOR

1. Get a commitment
2. Probe for supporting evidence
3. Reinforce what was done right
4. Correct mistakes
5. Teach a general rule

Allow the students to present what they know about the case, whether the situation involves an initial evaluation, deciding on a treatment plan, or progressing a rehabilitation. Asking the students to commit to an idea fosters their ownership of the problem because they will be accountable for the patient care decision. Prompting the students with open-ended questions such as, "What do you think is going on with this patient?" "What is your initial assessment?" and "What is your plan of care?" allows your students to articulate their thoughts and stimulates further questioning from the ACI.

The key to remember during this step of the OMP model is to accept the student's response in a nonthreatening manner. Appreciate that getting a commitment can be anxiety producing for some students.[3] In addition, be sure to listen for incorrect responses that may lead to a teaching opportunity.[3]

PROBE FOR SUPPORTING EVIDENCE

The next step in the OMP model is to probe for supporting evidence. This process allows you to explore the students' thought process and "diagnose" the learner's knowledge level. Probing questions that you might consider include the following:

- "What did you find in your exam that led you to your diagnosis?"
- "Were there any red flags in the patient's history?"
- "What can you do to rule out your differential diagnoses?"
- "What is your rationale for choosing those modality parameters?"
- "Now that you have talked through things, is there anything else you would like to do in your clinical exam?"

Some key points to remember when probing for evidence is that by allowing the student to think out loud you can assess his or her knowledge and decision-making process. You may need to use a leading question such as "Are there any contraindications for using a heating modality with this patient?" However, you should avoid leading questions that have a negative tone and that denigrate the student's thought process, such as, "Why didn't you ask the patient about his pain level?"

You should also allow the student ample time to collect his or her thoughts regarding his or her supporting rationale. You will find that students will become familiar with the OMP format and will anticipate your questions. This will motivate them to be more prepared in the clinical setting as they become more familiar with the type of patient information they need to present to the ACI during teachable moments.

While the first 2 micro-skills we have discussed should always occur in order, the last 3 skills may be interchanged depending on the situation.

REINFORCE WHAT WAS DONE RIGHT

It is very important to encourage correct behaviors so that they may be repeated in the future. Providing positive feedback is a critical step in not only reinforcing skills that are performed correctly but also in building students' self-esteem and clinical confidence. Feedback should be specific and focus on behaviors. You should avoid vague feedback such as, "You did a good job." By being more specific, such as, "You were correct to consider ruling out an MCL sprain," the student knows exactly what was performed correctly and is more likely to repeat the correct performance when working with future patients. You may find that reinforcing behaviors is also helpful after you get a commitment from the student. For example, during the commitment step, a student may present several differential diagnoses to you. It would certainly be appropriate to reinforce that it is correct to consider multiple options before probing for evidence on each differential diagnosis.

CORRECT MISTAKES

The OMP micro-skill of correcting mistakes often occurs simultaneously with reinforcing behaviors. These corrections can be initiated by both the ACI and the student. Students benefit from the opportunity to reflect on their performance. Therefore, it can be helpful to first ask the student to self-identify what he or she did well and what he or she needs to improve. Similar to reinforcing what went well, the ACI should provide corrective feedback that is specific. For example, telling a student, "You were right to rule out an MCL sprain, but remember that the medial meniscus could also be involved based on the mechanism of injury" is more useful than saying, "You forgot a few special tests."

TEACH A GENERAL RULE

The last micro-skill in the OMP model is teaching general rules. It is important here not to get bogged down in a mini lecture on a particular topic. Teach the student a few pearls that can be applied to future cases. For example, a general rule about therapeutic modalities you may share with the student could be, "Research tells us that early application of high volt stimulation in the first 24 hours can curb edema formation." This is a general rule that can be applied to future cases without diving into an in-depth lecture on the biochemical response to cathodal stimulation. Teaching general rules can also serve as a jumping off point to encourage students to do additional reading or review.

APPLICATION OF THE ONE-MINUTE PRECEPTOR

Now that you are familiar with the 5 steps of the OMP, let us see what it looks like in action. Table 10-2 illustrates a scenario utilizing the OMP model. Notice that the

TABLE 10-2

THE ONE-MINUTE PRECEPTOR IN ACTION

After baseball practice, the first baseman comes into the athletic training room complaining of shoulder pain.

ACI: "Why don't you (student) go ahead and take a look at him and then tell me what you think. I'll be right here watching." (NOTE: This student has already had a course in upper extremity evaluation and this is the first "real-time" shoulder evaluation.)

Junior Student: "Sounds good." The student completes an evaluation that is clearly incomplete and feels ready to report to the ACI.

ACI: "So what do you think is going on with him?" (Get a commitment)

Student: "Well, I think he has impingement syndrome."

ACI: "What did you find in your exam that led to that diagnosis?" (Probe for evidence)

Student: "He had a positive impingement test."

ACI: "Are there any other symptoms or findings in the patient's history to support your diagnosis?" (Probe for evidence)

Student: "Um, he said it hurts when he throws and it is a 6/10 on the pain scale."

ACI: "Well, you did a good job performing the impingement test." (Enforce what was done well) "Is there anything else you think you should do to help confirm your diagnosis?"

Student: "I didn't really ask enough history questions and I didn't think to look at his posture either."

ACI: "Good. I'm glad you recognized that you missed those components of the exam." (Correct mistakes) "Always remember that it is important to examine the scapulohumeral rhythm in shoulder patients as poor scapular stabilization can often be a contributing factor to impingement." (Teach a general rule).

ACI is giving the student the autonomy to attempt an evaluation while still providing an adequate level of supervision. The student obviously misses a few steps, but the ACI refrains from jumping in too soon and withholds feedback until the student is completely finished with the assessment. The student offers a commitment but clearly lacks supporting evidence for the clinical diagnosis. The ACI reinforces what the student did well and offers probing questions to make the student think about his or her performance. The student is able to constructively reflect on areas that need improvement, thus allowing the ACI to better "diagnose" the student's understanding of the injury evaluation process. The ACI teaches a general rule about the shoulder evaluation that can be applied in future injury and/or rehabilitation situations.

REFLECTION QUESTIONS

Draw your own insights about the OMP model for the following scenario and questions:

Scenario

During morning rehabilitation, the baseball player mentioned in Table 10-2 reports to the athletic training room for his first day of rehabilitation for his shoulder impingement. The senior student assigned to morning rehabilitation hours is eager to begin developing a rehabilitation plan for this patient.

ACI: "Why don't you go ahead and do a quick assessment and tell me where you think we should begin with his session today."

The student does a quick postural assessment and returns to the ACI.

ACI: "So what do you think our plan should be today?"

Student: "I think we should start with some tubing exercises and then 3 sets of 10 prone T-exercises with 10 pounds. Then he should do 3 sets of 15 overhand tosses on the plyoback tramp."

ACI: "Well, that is pretty aggressive when you haven't even identified what your goals are for the session. Why don't you back up and develop a list of problems we need to address for this patient?"

Student: (clearly deflated) "Oh, I guess I screwed that up."

ACI: "Maybe it would be a good idea for you to go back and review some shoulder rehabilitation protocols while I get the patient started."

- What do you observe in the scenario that was an appropriate illustration of the OMP?
- What areas need improvement?
- Develop specific suggestions to improve the teaching exchange.

Reflection

Reflect upon your own experience as an ACI and identify a clinical teaching exchange that you felt was not particularly effective. Discuss how the OMP model could be applied to improve that situation.

REFERENCES

1. Henning JM, Weidner TG. Role strain in collegiate athletic training approved clinical instructors. *J Athl Train*. 2008;43:275-283.
2. Neher JO, Gordon KC, Meyer B, Stevens N. A five-step "microskills" model of clinical teaching. *J Am Board Fam Pract*. 1992;5:419-424.
3. Kertis M. The one-minute preceptor: a five-step tool to improve clinical teaching. *J Nurs Staff Dev*. 2007;23:238-242.

11

Clinical Teaching for Various Clinical Settings and Situations

Thomas G. Weidner, PhD, ATC, FNATA

Certainly, there are more similarities than differences when it comes to clinical teaching across various settings and situations. However, important distinctions can arise. The purpose of this chapter is to help you gain an appreciation of some of the key distinctions to consider when serving as an approved clinical instructor (ACI) for students in common off-campus clinical settings (ie, outpatient rehabilitation clinic and high school). As well, clinical teaching during an on-the-field injury situation will also be addressed. Finally, real-time clinical experiences and case-based simulations for clinical teaching will be overviewed and recommended. See Appendix A regarding online clinical teaching resources that are intended to augment this chapter.

CLINICAL TEACHING IN THE OUTPATIENT REHABILITATION CLINIC AND HIGH SCHOOL SETTINGS

Rehabilitation clinic and high school sites are likely the most often utilized athletic training clinical education settings outside of the college/university athletic training room. CAATE accreditation standards[1] encourage clinical placements in such settings. In so doing, students become familiar with the essential distinctions and characteristics associated with these settings and more appreciative of the profession at-large. Such experiences can also provide students with invaluable opportunities to apply their knowledge and skills in new ways with different populations. The outcome of such is often increased student confidence, an aspect of professional preparation that tends to be highly challenging.

Clinical teaching in these settings should include an initial student orientation to his or her key distinctions. Clinical instructors would do well to then focus on these specific areas, including but not limited to the following suggestions:

- Accepting and appreciating the roles of allied health professionals.

- Providing education and guidance on preventative techniques specific to the patient population.

- Demonstrating injury evaluation and management skills for injuries/illnesses specific to the patient population.

- Utilizing proper treatment, rehabilitation, and reconditioning techniques for the injury/illness/condition specific to the patient population.

- Demonstrating an understanding of the organization, administration, marketing, and delivery of sports medicine care delivered in the rehabilitation clinic and high school settings.

- Demonstrating effective communication skills with patients and allied health professionals.

- Demonstrating an appreciation of diversity and age-group characteristics of the patient population served in the rehabilitation clinic and high school settings.

- Using clinical outcome assessments through clinician-based (eg, strength, ROM) or patient-based (eg, satisfaction, return to function) measures.

To the extent possible, the student could be held accountable to make certain that clinical experiences in these areas are completed. Learning activities in these settings could also incorporate medical abbreviations, SOAP notes, in-services for coaches or parents, and patient home instruction brochures or FAQs. See Appendix H for a sample of an online clinical experience update report (completed by students every 2 to 3 weeks) that could both guide and monitor clinical experiences and activities regarding these distinct areas. A corresponding online student clinical performance evaluation form (completed by the ACI mid-way and at completion of rotation) can also be found in Appendix I as well as further guides clinical experiences regarding these distinct areas. Clinical teaching for other settings (eg, industrial, military) could be fashioned and modeled after these examples.

CLINICAL TEACHING: ON-THE-FIELD INJURY SITUATION

A clinical teaching situation that is more complex because of urgency and/or imposed time constraints is the on-the-field injury. On-the-field injuries can be divided into ambulatory and athlete-down types.[2] Because ambulatory conditions are marked by the athlete's coming to the athletic trainer to be evaluated, there is little difference between ambulatory evaluation and clinical evaluation in the athletic training room. However, the amount of time available to perform the evaluation certainly may be decreased during competition. In an athlete-down situation, the athletic trainer may be confronted with a number of possible scenarios. In order of their importance, the on-field evaluation must rule out the following:[2]

- Inhibition of the cardiovascular and respiratory systems
- Life-threatening trauma to the head or spinal column
- Profuse bleeding
- Fractures
- Joint dislocation
- Peripheral nerve injury
- Other soft tissue trauma

Clinical teaching in athlete-down situations may be difficult and stressful at best. If feasible, and if ready, it may be that the student may take over during any of the steps above. Most likely, the ACI will give the student somewhat less independence initially, prompting and guiding the student through the process. Or perhaps, based on the findings of the triage completed by the athletic trainer and observed by the student, the student could then offer impressions of the condition and recommend the immediate disposition of the athlete. This would include suggestions regarding the on-field management of the injury, the safest method of removing the athlete from the field, and the urgency of referring the athlete for further medical care. In cases of head or spine trauma, perhaps the student could be responsible for stabilizing the spine while the athletic trainer performs the evaluation. It may also be that the student could be instructed to communicate with the sidelines through pre-established hand signals or walkie-talkies. The student should be familiar with the pertinent rules governing the administration of medical assistance during an athlete-down situation. Before a contest, the student should join the athletic trainer in meeting with the officials to clarify any points. Very significantly, and when time permits, debrief the student regarding the experience with the athlete-down situation. This could include inquiring about the student's knowledge of the evaluation steps and observations of what could have been done differently, as well as feelings resulting from such a situation. Ultimately, the more experiences a student has in assisting with on-the-field injuries, the more the student becomes desensitized to the incumbent special demands of managing a potential emergency situation in the future.

REAL-TIME LEARNING EXPERIENCES AND CASE-BASED SIMULATIONS

It is easy to appreciate that the application of clinical proficiencies (including for on-the-field injury situations) do not always occur at the right place and at the right time simply for the benefit of student learning.[3] Real-time clinical experiences are certainly valued as a hallmark process for professional growth,[4] as they occur at unpredictable times in unpredictable environments.[4] In real-time clinical experiences, students have the opportunity to apply theory into clinical practice, which includes integrating critical-thinking and decision-making processes.[4] Ideally, real-time clinical experiences need to be the top priority for clinical teaching as they allow students to make clinical decisions[4] that depend on identifying and understanding the clinical situation. In real-time experiences, students are more able to see the patient or the clinical situation and understand the significance of the patient's needs.[5] Unfortunately, a majority of the clinical proficiencies are not being applied during real-time clinical experiences.[6] Too often, students depend heavily on the ACI or choose not to use their time wisely, relying too much on simulated clinical proficiency evaluations.[3] ACIs and students need to capitalize on real-time situations whenever feasible. Student confidence regarding clinical abilities and mastery of clinical practice is enhanced through real-time encounters with patients.[4] More use of real-time clinical experiences in athletic training would aid in developing proficient and sensitive practitioners for the profession.

It is unlikely, however, that there will be sufficient overall opportunities for real-time clinical experiences because injuries/conditions will not always occur at the right place and at the right time. This supports the need for authentic alternative clinical experiences to help ensure that athletic training students have received adequate preparation for entry-level practice. Case-based simulations provide students with opportunities to apply and integrate clinical skills during a scenario with a mock patient/athlete. It is important to make clear here that such simulated experiences should not take a checklist approach to psychomotor skills and omit attention to communication abilities and professional behaviors.[4] Case-based simulations can enhance both clinical and reasoning skills.[7] This includes organizing information to be recalled later for use in clinical reasoning situations, generating experiences that students would not otherwise have, increasing the visibility of students' clinical reasoning processes, and enhancing students' confidence.

Clinical reasoning is enhanced by appropriate organization of knowledge. Problem-solving ability cannot be applied across clinical problems. Rather, clinical reasoning is context-dependent, specific to a presenting situation.[8] So even though athletic training students are becoming expert in one kind of clinical situation, they may be novices in unfamiliar situations.[9] Clinical reasoning actually incorporates both knowledge and cognitive processes. This means that organization of knowledge is crucial because, even though we are able to hold only a limited number of units or chunks of information for immediate memory, the amount of information can be increased through incorporating information into larger chunks.[10] Clinical reasoning requires considering many pieces of information that are organized for efficient recall and utilization. Students can particularly develop their expertise if they are assisted in learning and experiencing information in a way that parallels the way in which that information will be used and retrieved in the future. Case-based simulations provide structure and application of knowledge in a context-specific way.

Clinical assignments are intended to provide students with a range of experiences. However, certain opportunities for learning do not occur for all students. Gaps are a concern because of the importance of prototype cases for clinical reasoning. Proficient and expert clinicians develop clusters of prototype cases that they use in making judgments about particular clinical problems.[11] Simulated cases could be used to supplement and generate experiences that students would not otherwise have and to function as prototypical cases.

Student dialogue regarding a simulated case can expose students' critical-thinking, problem-solving, and clinical-reasoning processes. For instance, your students may focus on a part of a case and ignore other issues. This facilitates student and ACI assessment of learning needs. For instance, it may be that a poor patient history led to a poor presumptive diagnosis. The student and the ACI can now spend time reviewing the purposes and contents of a good history and its relationship to an accurate diagnosis.

Simulated cases also allow for clarification of misunderstandings and misinterpretations. Through continuing analysis, reasoning, and collaborating with the ACI regarding the case, the student can gain a sense of mastery and confidence that will grow with clinical experience[12] provided through case-based simulations, thus instilling a strong sense of personal efficacy.[13] Case-based simulation is therefore an important component of clinical education, filling in some of the experiences that may not be available in real time.

SAMPLE CASE-BASED SIMULATION

Case-based simulations can occur in a variety of ways. Typically, a peer or the ACI can serve as the mock patient/athlete. In down-time occasions during clinical experiences, the ACI may create a case that will be simulated (to the extent possible). For example, one athletic training student could be privately briefed (or initially quizzed) regarding the essential findings for diagnosis of an inversion ankle sprain. Following any necessary clarifications, the ACI and this student (mock athlete) could consider an injury case in which to portray/roleplay (eg, injury scenario, history regarding past injury, extent of symptoms, limping, amount of tenderness during palpations). At this point, another athletic training student would be instructed to evaluate the simulated case. This may begin with a set-up regarding the context of the situation (eg, down athlete on the field). As well, important ground rules should be explained, including instructions that the student should restrict the evaluation to only those items that are considered essential for diagnosis of the case at hand (including differentials). In other words, do not take a checklist approach by addressing all items that could possibly be included in an evaluation of the ankle joint. The ACI should also note that communication skills and professional behaviors during the evaluation of the case will be observed (to the extent feasible).

At the conclusion of the evaluation, the athletic training student should state the presumptive diagnosis and the other essential injuries that have been ruled out. This process could be guided by inquiring which information obtained during the history, observation, palpation, etc led to these conclusions. At this point, with what has been observed during the evaluation and the subsequent verbal description of what has been reasoned, the ACI has clear visibility of the student's clinical critical-thinking and problem-solving processes. Closure of the simulated case would now include dialogue regarding which skills and processes were done well and which could use some correction and redirection. Per the information presented in the previous section regarding the benefits of case-based simulations, this experience will promote clarification of misunderstandings, assessment of learning needs, and a greater sense of mastery and confidence for future cases. The simulated case can now also serve as a prototype for use in evaluation of similar cases.

As time and interest allow, authenticity and fidelity can be added to the simulated cases. For more acute injury situations, resources are available that could enhance the appearance of the actual injury (eg, prosthetic limbs, bleeding, swelling, discoloration). EMT training refers to this authentic replication as mallage. An Internet search of casualty simulation kits will yield such resources for the purpose. Perhaps less feasible for the clinician/ACI, but worth noting, is the use of standardized patients (SPs). A SP can be described as an individual who has undergone special training to more formally and consistently portray an injury or condition to multiple students. A standardized patient encounter is different than a simulated case in that a SP case must be carefully developed and the SP must be trained to accurately and consistently portray that case. Once the case is developed, a SP is found or recruited that fits the age, sex, and physical characteristics needed for the case. That individual then undergoes individual or group training with a SP trainer (an individual who is experienced or trained to work with SPs). Substantial evidence exists in the medical literature that SPs are widely accepted to assess the clinical competence and performance of medical students.[14,15] A recent literature review revealed the realism of SP encounters. Based on research where unannounced SPs were sent into physicians' offices, well-trained SPs are difficult to differentiate from real patients.[16] Over the past 30 years, SPs have been utilized in medical education to evaluate (and teach) clinical skills,[17] ensuring that students accurately and realistically experience a variety of clinical situations prior to practicing on actual patients. Recently, other allied health care professions such as nursing and physical therapy are beginning to investigate the impact of SPs in their professional preparation programs.

REFLECTION QUESTIONS

Draw your own insights about whether you are providing effective clinical teaching for various situations in your setting by answering these questions:

- What do you feel are the essential distinctions and characteristics associated with your setting that should receive specific attention during students' clinical experiences?

- What learning activities could be designed regarding the above areas? How could the learning activities be monitored/evaluated?

- How can you improve athletic training students' clinical experiences in athlete-down injury situations?

- How can real-time clinical experiences be improved in your setting?

- How can case-based simulations be incorporated into students' clinical experiences in your setting?

REFERENCES

1. Commission on Accreditation of Athletic Training Education. Standards for the accreditation of entry-level athletic training education programs. Available at http://caate.net/ss_docs/standards.6.8.2006. pdf. Accessed November 7, 2007.
2. Starkey C, Ryan JL. *Evaluation of Orthopedic and Athletic Injuries.* 2nd ed. Philadelphia, PA: F.A. Davis; 2002.
3. Armstrong KJ, Weidner TG, Walker SE. Athletic training approved clinical instructors are primarily using simulations for evaluating clinical proficiencies. *J Athl Train.* In press.
4. Cullen DL. Clinical education and clinical evaluation of respiratory therapy students. *Respir Care Clin N Am.* 2005;11(3):425-447.
5. White AH. Clinical decision making among fourth-year nursing students: an interpretive study. *J Nurs Educ.* 2003;42(3):113-120.
6. Walker SE, Weidner TG, Armstrong KJ. Athletic training students' clinical proficiencies are primarily evaluated via simulations. *J Athl Train.* 2008;43(4):386-395.
7. Thomas MD, O'Connor FW, Albert ML, Boutain D, Brandt PA. Case-based teaching and learning experiences. *Issues Mental Health Nurs.* 2001;22:517-531.
8. Mandin H, Jones A, Woloschuk W, Harasym P. Helping students learn to think like experts when solving clinical problems. *Acad Med.* 1997;72(3):173-179.
9. Benner P. *From Novice to Expert: Excellence and Power in Clinical Nursing Practice.* Menlo Park, CA: Addison-Wesley; 1984.
10. Miller GA. The magical number seven plus or minus two: some limits on our capacity for processing information. *Psychol Rev.* 1956;63(2):81-97.
11. Fowler LP. Clinical reasoning strategies used during care planning. *Clin Nurs Res.* 1997;6(4):349-361.
12. Radwin LE. Empirically generated attributes of experience in nursing. *J Adv Nurs.* 1998;27(3):590-595.
13. Bandura A. Personal and collective efficacy in human adaptation and change. In: Adair JG, Belanger D, Dion KL, eds. *Advances in Psychological Sciences. Vol 1. Social, Personal, and Cultural Aspects.* East Sussex, UK: Psychology Press; 1998:51-71.
14. Ebbert DW, Connors H. Standardized patient experiences: evaluation of clinical performance and nurse practitioner student satisfaction. *Nurse Educ Prospect.* 2004;25:12-15.
15. Norcini J, Boulet J. Methodological issues in the use of standardized patients for assessment. *Teach Learn Med.* 2003;15(4):293.
16. Boulet JR, De Champlain AF, McKinley DW. Setting defensible performance standards on OSCEs and standardized patient examinations. *Med Teach.* 2003;25:245-249.
17. Weidner TG, Henning JM. Historical perspective of athletic training clinical education. *J Athl Train.* 2002;37(4 Suppl):S222-S228.

SECTION III

CLOSING THE LOOP

Evaluation and Feedback
Keys to Clinical Success

Thomas G. Weidner, PhD, ATC, FNATA

The primary goal of athletic training clinical education is to help students acquire, develop, and master clinical proficiencies.[1] These clinical proficiencies list the content areas, skills, and knowledge necessary for an entry-level athletic trainer.[2] Thus, successfully developing these clinical proficiencies must be a significant focus of students' clinical experience,[3] and approved clinical instructors (ACIs) must be accountable for teaching, documenting, and evaluating clinical proficiencies.

Accurate assessment of student clinical skills is a key issue for all health profession educators. Student clinicians must reliably perform the skills correctly and safely on real-life patients before they can enter a professional practice, and the consumer public requires assurance that students can achieve and/or exceed a minimum standard of care.[4] Additionally, evaluation provides academic and clinical information regarding student progress, enabling ACIs to assign student grades, to determine whether students have attained entry-level competence, and to help assess the overall effectiveness of the academic and clinical curricula.[5]

In allied health professions education, feedback is also necessary for teaching students appropriate patient care.[6] Appropriate feedback helps students correct their mistakes, reinforces good performance, and maintains clinical competence.[6] This chapter will describe and overview specific methods of clinical proficiency evaluation and feedback, including self-evaluation and peer evaluation.

WHAT ABOUT EVALUATION?

As an ACI, you will note athletic training students' knowledge, skills, and behaviors as they relate to the specific goals and objectives of their clinical experience. This will include noting student progress during the clinical experience based on performance criteria established by the athletic training education program (ATEP). You will identify areas of competence as well as areas that require improvement. Students want and need to know how they are performing, so you will need to approach this evaluation process as constructive and educational. Often, you will formally evaluate a student's performance at the middle and end of an educational experience in order to determine a grade. For example, many ACIs routinely complete clinical performance assessment questionnaires for each student with whom they have worked. Such questionnaires typically ask ACIs to rate the student's abilities, knowledge, and attitudes on a scale ranging from unsatisfactory to good or exceptional. This type of evaluation—summative evaluation—is important, but effective clinical teaching requires formative evaluation as well.[7]

Formative evaluation involves continuously providing feedback to students regarding how they are performing the tasks expected of them. This type of evaluation is intended to reinforce good performance or redirect and correct specific deficiencies. It is analogous to coaching in that it is an ongoing process of correction and reinforcement that helps shape desired performance and attitude. Formative evaluation also helps students evaluate their own knowledge and understanding, identify strengths and weaknesses without incurring academic penalty, and understand the expectations of the ACI. Providing formative evaluation encourages interaction between the ACI and athletic training student, helps to build a productive working and learning relationship between the two, and is a means for expressing interest in and concern for the progress and development of the student.[7] Effective ACIs use multiple sources of assessment in order to capture and/or confirm a student's clinical performance (eg, clinical experience update reports, observation of the student's performance of various tasks, conversations with patients and staff). If an athletic training student needs remediation, the ACI needs to communicate with the program director and/or clinical education coordinator in a timely manner. The ACI should also communicate to program administrators any problems with performance evaluation instruments.[8]

WHAT IS FEEDBACK? WHY IS IT IMPORTANT?

Feedback is information used to make adjustments in reaching a goal.[6] It occurs when a student is given insight by the ACI into what he or she actually did as well as the consequences of that action. In giving feedback, the ACI serves as the mirror, providing information to the student about the desired behavior, the actual observed behavior, and any dissonance that might exist between the two. Feedback is not judgmental in nature. It presents information that helps the student reach clinical experience objectives and develop expertise in the care of patients.

PROVIDING EFFECTIVE FEEDBACK[6,9]

1. Rapport: Establish a relationship with the student in which effective learning and improved patient care are central. Find a quiet, private, comfortable place for communicating feedback.

2. Timing: Provide feedback often and as soon after the event being evaluated as possible. Make feedback a regular, natural part of the clinical experience.

3. Content:
   o Begin by soliciting the student's thoughts on his or her performance (eg, "How do you think it went? What aspects of the patient encounter were successful?").

o It is important to give positive and constructive comments focused on behaviors that can be changed. A behavior embedded in a personality trait would be difficult to resolve.

o Sandwich negative feedback between positive comments about performance. Suggest correct performance rather than emphasizing what was done wrong (eg, "Next time, try..."). Focus on decisions and behaviors rather than individual abilities or traits (eg, "A better therapy choice here would be..." rather than, "Your knowledge of therapies seems inadequate.").

o Limit the quantity of feedback given at any one time.

o Ask the student to explain the feedback given (eg, "Would you summarize what you will do when you see this patient in follow-up next week?").

4. Patient care: Patients also can be asked to give feedback to students after a clinical encounter. Skills that are especially appropriate for patients to address include the following:

o Did the student encourage the patient to express personal concerns?

o Did the student listen to the patient's concerns?

o Did the student treat patients with respect?

o Did the student present information clearly and appropriately?

o Did the student treat patients as partners in their care?[10]

PROMOTING CONTINUOUS EVALUATION

By making feedback a natural part of the learning and practice environment, you can help students adopt the habit of self-evaluation and continuous, lifelong learning. ACIs can use techniques to promote this self-evaluation. In addition to continually giving feedback to students, ACIs can model how to listen to and receive feedback, for instance, by asking students about the usefulness of various aspects of the clinical learning experience and helpful and hindering ACI behaviors.

Enlisting others in the clinical environment to provide feedback to students can help to build a more comprehensive and intensive learning environment. In addition, it can help accustom students to accepting and using feedback about their performance on a continual basis to improve their practice. For example, you may recognize that one of your students now seems to be improving in taking an injury history.

Another way to promote continuous evaluation is through self-evaluation. Set explicit performance standards with students and have them regularly evaluate themselves in comparison with those standards.[7] Appendix I is an example of a clinical performance self-evaluation instrument. Students could complete this mid-way through a clinical assignment and consider ways to strengthen their performance for the remainder of the clinical assignment. ACIs could simultaneously evaluate their students with basically this same instrument and both completed instruments could be compared and contrasted during a discussion with the students.

Peer evaluation provides yet another forum for feedback. If several students are present in the office or athletic training room, they can be encouraged to provide feedback to one another through discussion of various aspects of patient care. Research suggests that students learn at a deeper level when they teach their peers[11,12] and seem to have a higher level of self-awareness of their own skill level when they evaluate their peers.[13] Peer evaluation is an especially effective tool for enhancing athletic training students' comprehension and performance of clinical psychomotor skills,[13,14] targeting those skills that may be part of a proficiency but not the clinical proficiency itself (eg, stress test for the knee, but not the entire knee evaluation). Thus, peer evaluation supplements, rather than replaces, ACI instruction and evaluation (see Chapter 8 regarding peer-assisted learning and ways to implement peer evaluation in athletic training education).

EVALUATION OF CLINICAL PROFICIENCIES

The fourth edition of the athletic training educational competencies, which contains the clinical proficiencies for effective preparation of the entry-level athletic trainer, defines proficient as "performing with expert correctness and facility."[2] Because clinical proficiencies measure real-life application, successfully developing these content areas must represent a significant focus of the students' clinical experience and be organized in such a way that faculty and staff of the ATEP can evaluate and monitor student progress over time.[2,3]

If the goal of clinical education is to aid in the acquisition, development, and mastery of clinical proficiencies,[1] then it is important to evaluate clinical proficiencies similarly to the ways they will be applied in real life. Performance-based assessment is intimately linked to professional practice, where the performance being assessed must reflect and represent the real-life practice of the profession.[15] Although a certified athletic trainer (ATC) is considered competent upon passing the Board of Certification (BOC) exam,[16] current testing methods do not necessarily evaluate clinical proficiencies, leaving this important responsibility chiefly with the accredited ATEPs and their ACIs.[3]

Research with ATEPs and ACIs indicates that athletic training students' clinical proficiencies are primarily being evaluated via simulations,[17,18] defined as a scenario or clinical situation in which a student evaluates a mock patient/athlete who portrays an injury or condition (eg, shoulder pain, acute cervical spine injury). The mock patient/athlete, typically a peer student or ACI, has had no training to portray the injury or condition in a standardized and consistent fashion. A vast majority (93%) of the ATEPs reported utilizing simulations at some point to evaluate clinical proficiencies.[17] Further, these simulations were used more than 50% of the time to evaluate clinical proficiencies by a little over half of the ATEPs.

Real-time clinical proficiency evaluation was defined as when an athletic training student was directly engaged with an actual patient/athlete. Although a majority of ATEPs (92%) reported that clinical proficiencies are evaluated in real time, only 24% reported that real-time evaluations of clinical proficiencies are used more than half of the time.[17] At least half of those responding would prefer more real-time clinical proficiency evaluations for their students. Regardless of preference or number of clinical hours, however, real-time opportunities are unpredictable, and so ACIs must use simulations in order to evaluate clinical proficiencies. As is the case in medical clinical education, athletic training students' real-time clinical proficiency evaluation and instruction are limited by the timely occurrence of an injury/condition. Respondents felt that the following clinical content areas often provided real-time experience for students[17,18]:

- Orthopedic clinical examination and diagnosis
- Therapeutic modalities

- Conditioning and rehabilitative exercise
- Risk management and injury prevention.
- In contrast, these content areas were felt to provide insufficient real-time opportunities:
- Nutritional aspects of injury and illness
- Psychosocial intervention and referral content areas[17,18]

ACIs' willingness or availability to complete real-time clinical proficiency evaluations may particularly impact the incidence of this method of evaluation. Over half of the respondents indicated that patient/athlete health care is more often a priority over student clinical education.[17,18] Perhaps clinical proficiency evaluation could be improved if ACIs were to proactively take advantage of real-time opportunities.

REFLECTION QUESTIONS

Draw your own insights about whether you are providing effective evaluation and feedback for your students by answering these questions:

- What can you do as an ACI to provide students with both formative and summative evaluation while under your supervision?
- What strategies can you employ as an ACI to provide quality feedback to a student?
- What strategies or techniques can you personally employ for listening to and receiving feedback?
- How could you use multiple students at one clinical education experience to provide feedback to one another?
- What can you do as an ACI to encourage and promote real-time evaluation of clinical proficiencies?

REFERENCES

1. Cheung MT, Yau KK. Objective assessment of a surgical trainee. *ANZ J Surg*. 2002;72(5):325-330.
2. National Athletic Trainers' Association. *Athletic Training Educational Competencies*. 4th ed. Dallas, TX: Author; 2006.
3. Commission on Accreditation of Athletic Training Education. Standards for the accreditation of entry-level athletic training education programs. Available at: http://caate.net/ss_docs/standards.6.8.2006.pdf. Accessed November 7, 2007.
4. Allery L. How to assess trainees in the clinical workplace using Mini-CEX (mini clinical evaluation exercise). *Education for Primary Care*. 2006;17:240-244.
5. Campbell SK. Development of psychomotor objectives for classroom of clinical education in physical therapy. *Phys Ther*. 1977;57(9):1031-1034.
6. Ende J. Feedback in clinical medical education. *JAMA*. 1983;250(6):777-781.
7. FISPE Project Group. Evaluating performance and providing feedback. The Expert Preceptor Interactive Curriculum. Available at: http://www.med.unc.edu/epic/. Accessed July 13, 2005.
8. Weidner TG, Henning JM. Development of standards and criteria for the selection, training, and evaluation of athletic training approved clinical instructors. *J Athl Train*. 2004;39(4):335-343.
9. Stritter FT, Baker RM, Shahady EJ. Clinical instruction. In: McGaghie WC, Frey JJ, eds. *Handbook for the Academic Physician*. New York: Springer-Verlag; 1986.
10. Westberg J, Jason H. *Collaborative Clinical Education*. New York: Springer-Verlag; 1993.
11. Knight KL. Assessing *Clinical Proficiencies in Athletic Training: A Modular Approach*. 3rd ed. Champaign, IL: Human Kinetics; 2001.

12. Topping K. Peer assessment between students in colleges and universities. *Rev Educ Res.* 1998;68(3):249-276.

13. Topping K. *Peer-Assisted Learning: A Practical Guide for Teachers.* Newton, MA: Brookline Books; 2001.

14. Henning JM, Weidner TG, Jones J. Peer-assisted learning in the athletic training clinical setting. *J Athl Train.* 2006;41(1):102-108.

15. Munoz LQ, O'Bryne C, Pugsley J, Austin Z. Reliability, validity, and generalizability of an objective stuctured clinical examination (OSCE) for assessment of entry-to-practice in pharmacy. *Pharm Educ.* 2005;5(1):33-43.

16. Board of Certification. BOC 2005 testing report. Available at: http://www.bocatc.org/BOCATC_Files/bocweb/_Items/SI-MR-TAB8-436/docs/2005%20Annual%20Report%20%20on%20the%20Exam.pdf#search=%22BOCATC%20testing%20results%202005%22. Accessed December 18, 2006.

17. Walker SE, Weidner TG, Armstrong KJ. Evaluation of athletic training students' clinical proficiencies. *J Athl Train.* 2008;43(4):386-395.

18. Armstrong KJ, Weidner TG, Walker SE. Athletic training approved clinical instructors primarily utilize simulations for evaluating clinical proficiencies. *J Athl Train.* In press.

Dealing With the Difficult Learning Situation

Thomas G. Weidner, PhD, ATC, FNATA

This material was developed by the MAHEC Office of Regional Primary Care Education, Asheville, North Carolina and has been adapted with permission.

The vast majority of learning encounters proceed smoothly with significant benefit for the student and often a sense of reward and accomplishment for you as the ACI. But not always. Information in this chapter will help you to prevent potential problems and to deal more effectively with problems when they occur. This chapter is designed to accomplish the following:

- Help you to detect potential problems in the early stages
- Introduce an organized approach to assessing and managing challenging teacher/ student interactions
- Review a strategy to prevent problem interactions

DEALING WITH THE DIFFICULT LEARNING SITUATION: PREVENTION

The old adage "an ounce of prevention is worth a pound of cure" is as true in clinical teaching as it is in athletic training. It is generally much more efficient (and pleasant) to prevent a problem than to manage the negative impact once it has occurred. In athletic training, as in education, there are different kinds of prevention: primary, secondary, and tertiary (Table 13-1). Primary prevention seeks to avoid the problem before it occurs. The goal in secondary prevention is early detection and decisive action. Tertiary prevention is the management of existing problems in order to minimize the negative impact of those problems. Each level of prevention has its own characteristics and strengths.

TABLE 13-1

PREVENTION

PRIMARY: PREVENT THE PROBLEM BEFORE IT OCCURS

- Know the learning objectives for the clinical experience course.
- Orient the student well.
- Set clear expectations and goals.
- Determine the student's own goals and expectations.
- Reassess mid-course.

SECONDARY: EARLY DETECTION

- Pay attention to your hunches/clues.
- Do not wait.
- Initiate SOAP early.
- Give specific feedback early and monitor closely.

TERTIARY: MANAGE A PROBLEM TO MINIMIZE IMPACT

- If it is not working, seek help.
- Do not be a martyr.
- Do not give a passing grade to a student who has not earned it.

Primary Prevention

As in athletic training, the prevention of problems or issues before they occur is the ideal. Fortunately, there are several strategies that can help prevent difficult teacher/student interactions. Expectations must be clear:

- What does the athletic training education program (ATEP) expect of this clinical experience?
- What does the student expect from this experience?
- What do you as the ACI expect of the student?

As the ACI, you will need to know the specific expectations for the learning experience. Some experiences may not be specific, allowing you wide latitude in structuring the clinical placement. Other experiences may delineate highly specific learning objectives for the student. Become acquainted with any specific expectations before you agree to accept the placement, and review those expectations with students at the beginning.

An important step in any clinical rotation is to fully orient the student to your specific site, including clearly explaining what you expect. What time does he or she need to arrive? What are the weekend expectations? What format do you prefer in documentation? What is your dress code? These and many other issues can vary significantly from site to site and should be specifically addressed with the student from the beginning. A clear understanding of your expectations and goals can help the student adapt to your environment and avoid significant problems.

Students also bring their own expectations to a placement or learning experience. They may expect a certain level of responsibility or clinical experiences that are not available in your practice situation. Detecting any mismatches early can allow you to negotiate options before problems develop. By the same token, knowing the student's individual desires and goals will help you to make this a more successful experience for his or her.

Even if effective orientation and discussion occur at the beginning of the rotation, new or unanticipated issues can develop for the ACI and the student once the rotation is underway. Sitting down together halfway through the rotation creates an opportunity to reassess and refine goals and expectations for both the ACI and the student, setting the stage for an even smoother second half of the experience.

Secondary Prevention

If primary prevention has not succeeded, then early detection of problems is essential. The parallel with athletic training practice continues. As a clinician, you know that carefully observing, for instance, faulty mechanics or muscle imbalance can help you manage, and sometimes prevent, injury. The same principle holds true in teaching. Identify problems early in order to reduce the negative impact.

The secondary prevention outlined in Table 13-1 depends on maintaining awareness that things can go wrong. ACIs are often optimistic in dealing with their students. You have come to expect high-quality students with whom you are able to interact with in a positive and pleasant way. As a result, ACIs may ignore early warning signs, shrugging them off as "stress" or "a bad day." Pay close attention to any hunches or feelings that things may not be quite right. Additional clues can come from the comments or opinions of staff or partners. For example, when a staff member who has previously interacted well with other students begins to comment negatively on a current student in the setting, this could be an important warning sign. Every "red flag" (or even yellow flag) should be evaluated, just as attention should be paid to abnormal biomechanics. Intentional and frequent assessment of possible warning signs can help you pinpoint significant issues and address or ignore insignificant ones.

You may want to bide your time, observing: "Well, maybe this is a problem but it's just the first week and we've been kind of busy." In the clinical education setting, you must examine and address potential issues as early as possible due to the limited time of the contact. "Wait and see" can be costly and ineffective in a short educational experience. Plan to institute an organized assessment of a potential problem situation early, such as the "SOAP" method introduced later in this chapter. The earlier you begin looking critically at a situation, the more likely the student will succeed.

When a problem appears minor, you can give specific feedback on the issue to the student and then watch carefully to see if that feedback is acted upon. For example, let us say a third-year athletic training student is beginning a practicum in your clinical setting. During the first week you have noted that the student takes a much longer time in evaluating patients than previous students. You arrange a meeting with the student to review his performance (using specific examples). You also give specific suggestions, including time management with patients. You closely monitor the student's performance for the next 2 days in the clinical setting.

This "screening test" helps you to identify a problem behavior and intervene in a simple, unintrusive way to determine if the problem truly exists, but you have not formally assessed it. The key step is the follow-up. Closely monitor the situation for a limited time. If there is no longer a problem, then only continued monitoring is needed. If the problem behavior remains, then you need to make a careful assessment as soon as possible. Note that this is a different strategy from "wait and see." A brief active intervention is made and a brief period of observation follows, minimizing the chance of problem issues slipping through undetected. The judicious use of quality feedback and close follow-up is invaluable.

Tertiary Prevention

Sometimes in clinical education, as in patient care, a significant problem can arise despite the best efforts and intentions of the ACI and the ATEP. This is not a personal defeat or failure. Program administrators know that there will be an occasional difficult situation and are prepared and ready to assist you. Seeking help early and discussing concerns with a knowledgeable colleague can often ameliorate the situation.

Avoid the temptation to "just stick it out for a few more weeks." This does nothing to alleviate the negative impact of the problem on you, your staff, or your patients, and does not help the student. If you have been trying all the tricks and techniques that you know and are still not making any headway, then it is time to get help.

You do not need to be a martyr. ACIs often feel that they have made a commitment to work with the student through the entire rotation or experience no matter what. However, it is important to recognize a significantly negative situation and to seek help as needed to manage it. You are more valuable to the ATEP, your profession, and future students if you seek help early rather than burn out over one bad experience.

If you do not feel a student has earned a passing grade, do not pass that student. Athletic trainers must govern themselves. Thus, as a professional, you have a duty to avoid passing along a student who may not be able to serve the profession well. Communicate your concerns to the program director or other contact person for the ATEP in order to decide an appropriate course of action. Some grade choices may be available, such as "low pass" or "incomplete." Whatever the grade, it should be what the student earned, accurately reflecting the student's performance and abilities.

Summary

Some preventive measures that can help you to avoid many potentially difficult situations:

- Clearly set and communicate your expectations from the beginning
- Provide thoughtful, on-going feedback and evaluation throughout the student's rotation
- Pay attention to subtle clues

SOAP: AN APPROACH TO PROBLEM INTERACTIONS

You have paid attention to early warning signs and, despite your best efforts, you think there is a problem. How do you begin? Consider the SOAP format. This approach, adapted from Quirk,[1] is outlined in Table 13-2. In a step-by-step fashion it allows you to work from basic data to objective assessments to a differential diagnosis and a plan of action.

TABLE 13-2

SOAP: An Approach to Problem Interactions

SUBJECTIVE

- What do you/others think and say?

OBJECTIVE

- What are the specific behaviors that are observed?

ASSESSMENT

- Your differential diagnosis of the problem.

PLAN

- Gather more data? Intervene? Get help?

Subjective

In assessing a potential difficult ACI/student interaction, the subjective is usually "chief complaint." What was it that made you consider that there may be a problem with this student? Often an informal "label" assigned by you or someone in the setting may indicate a problem—"slow," "uninterested," "angry," "lazy."

Once you have a "chief complaint," then the history should be fleshed out. What do others in the setting think of this student and his or her performance during clinical experiences? Staff members who have had experience with several students can be insightful assessors of students' interpersonal skills, as students may act differently toward staff or patients than toward the ACI who will be grading them. Obtain data from all readily available sources and then determine if a pattern of behavior exists.

Another source of data is the student. A simple question about how he or she feels things are going may reveal that the student is aware of an issue and is working to remedy it. For example, if a student seems to be developing a habit of showing up late, you might ask, "How are things going with the rotation? I've noticed that you have been late a couple of times this week." This way, you give the student a chance to apologize and explain. If the student is unaware of the tardiness or unwilling to admit to it, you can more directly address the problem behavior.

These labels and impressions should not be considered the diagnosis of the problem. Just as fever is a symptom of an underlying condition, these impressions or descriptions may be symptoms of a more specific underlying diagnosis. In teaching, as in clinical practice, it is important not just to recognize and treat symptoms but to determine and act on an appropriate diagnosis. More specific information will be needed.

Objective

Once you have gathered information regarding a general pattern of behavior, you can identify and list specific examples. It is vitally important to be able to describe specific instances of problem behavior to the student. Students who are unaware of actions or attitudes likely to trigger a concern may have difficulty reviewing their performance to determine exactly what behaviors or episodes are responsible. You will need specific information to intervene effectively.

The following are examples of specific behaviors that you might list:

- "More than 20 minutes late on Monday, Tuesday, and Thursday this week."
- "Visit Thursday morning with Joe White: Took 40 minutes to assess this patient with a blister."
- "Spoke harshly to a fellow student when asking him to remind an athlete to make a return visit."
- "Unable to recall info on symptoms of meniscal injury on Wednesday AM after we had reviewed it on Tuesday."

A list of specific behaviors and specific instances of behavior (preferably written down) will help you to assess the nature of the problem, and later to decide on and initiate your plan of action.

Assessment

The next challenge is to analyze the information from the subjective and objective parts of your assessment and to consider possible causes—to work from the symptoms and manifestations of the problem to determine a diagnosis. As a trained clinician, you routinely consider a wide range of possible explanations for a physical condition. Likewise, as an ACI, you must also assess learning situations. Just as the clinical students you teach often produce short and incomplete differentials for clinical problems, ACIs sometimes come up short in assessing potential sources of learning difficulties. As with clinical practice, confidence and competence improve with experience. A guide to potential diagnoses for difficult ACI/student interactions is listed in Table 13-3.

Cognitive

One diagnostic category for learning difficulties is the cognitive area. If the student's knowledge base or skill base seems less than what you have come to expect for a student at a specific level, it may reflect a true deficit in his or her preparation. However, it may simply indicate that the student's knowledge is different from what you can actually expect at a given level. Students with different levels of training will certainly have markedly different levels of knowledge and clinical skills. Another explanation is that the student may have a learning disability. For instance, dyslexia, spatial perception problems, communication skill deficits, and attention deficit disorder have all been recognized in medical students. It is conceivable that a student in a demanding professional training program may have a learning disorder that has gone unrecognized, or a student who copes effectively in the classroom may find that the same strategies do not work in the clinical learning environment.

Finally, simple apathy may be behind a seemingly unprepared student's failure to perform well. A student oriented towards a different setting or career may not be highly motivated to excel in your setting. However, this should be a diagnosis of exclusion, a last resort after you have considered and excluded all other reasonable possibilities. Otherwise, you may miss an important issue (such as an undiagnosed learning disability).

Affective

A second diagnostic category includes affective or emotion-related concerns. New learning situations frequently result in significant initial nervousness and anxiety, but severe anxiety or nervousness can markedly affect performance. To differentiate

TABLE 13-3

ASSESSMENT—DIFFERENTIAL DIAGNOSIS

COGNITIVE

- Cognitive knowledge base/clinical skills less than expected?
- Dyslexia?
- Spatial perception difficulties?
- Communication difficulties?
- Lack of effort/interest?

AFFECTIVE

- Affective anxiety?
- Anger?
- Depression?

VALUATIVE

- Expects less work?
- Expects higher grade?
- Does not value specific rotation?
- Does not like your setting?
- Does not value your teaching?
- Holds principles that conflict with those held by you or your patients?

MEDICAL

- Recent illness?
- Chronic condition in poor control?
- Eating disorder?
- Substance abuse?
- Clinical depression?
- Anxiety/panic disorder?

between normal and extreme nervousness, observe the student for a few days. Is the student anxious only in specific situations, or is it a more generalized problem? Is the nervousness subsiding as the student becomes familiar with your setting? Does the student respond to reassurance and encouragement by relaxing more? Does the student's performance suffer as a result of anxiety? Normal nervousness will lessen with familiarity; persistent or severe anxiety should not be ignored. Further, a student's prior negative learning experiences may severely impair open communication with you. A beginning student may be intimidated by patient contact, as well. Perhaps the student is afraid of appearing too young or inexperienced. Perhaps the student is overwhelmed by the prospect of performing a physical exam on a real patient, a logical enough fear for a new professional. Students (and practicing clinicians) can sometimes be compromised in their work by the fear that they will harm a patient.

Anger is an emotion that compromises relationships. Unfortunately, students sometimes carry underlying prejudices or biases toward certain ethnic, social, or religious groups. Sometimes students have a superior attitude toward staff and assistants, or perhaps a student is angry at not having been assigned to a preferred clinical site. It is important to recognize anger and assess underlying causes early.

Depression can also severely affect performance, including a normal response to a life situation (ie, returning to school after a recent death in the family or a miscarriage). Patience, compassion, and humor are appropriate here. See the section below for the more serious medical issue of clinical depression.

One strategy for determining if an affective diagnosis is present is to consider what emotion the student or learning situation produces in you. Do you feel anxious or nervous when you talk to the student? Are you sad or depressed after a day of working together? The affect the student produces in you can be an important clue to the affect of the student.

Valuative

The most common difficulties that arise in clinical education settings come under the valuative category of diagnoses. These problem situations usually result from a mismatch between the values and expectations of the student and those of the ACI. A student may not value your area of expertise, setting an uneasy tone from the outset. A student may allow personal or religious principles to enter into discussion with staff and patients, leading to conflict. A student may anticipate a lighter workload or an easy A, then feel resentful to discover longer hours and hard grading. By being aware and proactive early on (ie, thorough orientation, review of expectations, mid-rotation review), you can prevent many of these issues and enhance your students' learning experiences.

Medical

At times, a medical diagnosis may be at the root of an educational issue. A recent illness such as mononucleosis or pneumonia may affect performance. A chronic condition such as diabetes or asthma may occasionally interfere with a student's performance. Clinical depression or anxiety/panic disorder may occur occasionally as well, and some students will invariably suffer from eating disorders, substance abuse, or other addictive behaviors that can impede performance.

Assessing learning difficulties, whether they are cognitive, affective, valuative, or medical, may be a little out of your comfort zone, but remember 2 important facts:

1. As a health care provider, you are trained to make diagnoses. The same skills you use to develop a differential diagnosis on a patient may work with learning difficulties.

2. Help may be available even without a diagnosis in hand.

Plan

After you determine that a difficult situation exists, collect subjective and objective data and develop some sense of a possible diagnosis, your next step is to decide on a plan. Your plan of action must be highly dependent on the impact of the situation on you, your practice, and the student. See Table 13-4 for possible courses of action.

TABLE 13-4

PLAN

GATHER MORE DATA?

- Observe and record
- Discuss with student
- Contact ATEP

INTERVENE?

- Detailed behavior/specific feedback
- Specific recommendations for change
- Set interval for re-evaluation

GET HELP?

- Get assistance from ATEP
- Transfer student

Gather More Data?

In a mild situation with minimal negative impact, you may want to gather more data. This data will be of value in planning your own intervention or in communicating your concerns to the ATEP.

Consider discussing the issue with the student. Even at an early stage in your assessment of the situation, this could shed additional light on the issue, including the student's awareness of the issue and its potential causes.

You may want to contact the ATEP at this point, even for what appears to be a relatively minor concern. The ATEP can be a source of excellent advice and guidance as well as moral support and may have information from other settings/experiences that may shed light on your concerns.

Intervene?

You may be able to intervene within your setting if the difficult learning situation minimally impacts practice, staff, or patients. You might be able to remedy a valuative or mild affective issue by giving specific feedback. Your detailed observations will clarify areas of concern for the student and will allow you to make specific recommendations for change. Determine a set interval for reassessment to discuss improvements. Many students will make dramatic improvements by acting on your feedback. If an intervention is not successful, the problem may be larger than you had thought and help may be required.

Get Help?

As in clinical practice, an important first step is to carefully consider the seriousness of the situation and then decide on an appropriate plan. Just as you would not treat certain injuries without referring to a physician, you must assess which issues can be appropriately addressed in your setting. As a health care professional, you

TABLE 13-5

ISSUES THAT MAY AFFECT CLINICAL TEACHING

PERSONAL/PROFESSIONAL

- Health issues—personal, family
- Practice issues—staffing, over-scheduling, financial issues
- Relationship issues—personality clash

IMPORTANT QUESTIONS

- Can you do what you need to do with the student there?
- Do your issues seriously affect the student's education?

have a strong desire to help others and to solve their problems. Nonetheless, your relationship with the student is not a provider/patient relationship, but a teacher/student relationship. As mentioned earlier, contact with the ATEP can result in additional information that could help you in selecting an appropriate intervention.

The primary responsibility for the well-being of the student rests with the ATEP administrator, who likely has significant resources to help students in need. In some cases, it may be best to transfer a student to another setting in order for the student to thrive.

DEALING WITH THE DIFFICULT LEARNING SITUATION: APPROVED CLINICAL INSTRUCTOR ISSUES

To this point we have focused on issues related to the student. There are times when difficult student situations can occur due to ACI-related issues (Table 13-5). Personal illness or illness in family members may affect your ability to teach effectively. Sudden loss of a partner or key staff member can markedly affect an ACI's ability to serve the needs of a student. Unexpected financial or schedule-related pressures could upset a previously planned learning/teaching experience. At times, an unanticipated personality clash with a student will make it impossible to establish the necessary close working relationship of the student and ACI. When/if ACI issues occur, ask these 2 questions:

1. Is the student's presence preventing you from doing what you need to do?

2. Are your issues seriously affecting the education of the student?

The commitment to teach is a serious one, and sometimes we tend to ignore problems and their impact rather than declining to take a scheduled student. The result of this could be a lose/lose situation for the ACI and the student.

REFLECTION QUESTIONS

Draw your own insights about whether you are providing effective prevention and management of difficult learning situations by answering these questions:

- In what ways could you improve the systematic prevention of difficult learning situations?
- In what ways could you improve your assessment of challenging teacher/student interactions?
- In what ways could you improve your management of challenging teacher/student interactions?
- What potential mismatches (student/staff/patients/ACI) would lead you to contact the ATEP to consider potential dismissal of the student?
- What type of personal situations for you as the ACI would lead you to cancel a scheduled rotation for a student?

REFERENCE

1. Quirk ME. *How to Teach and Learn in Medical School.* Springfield, IL: Charles C. Thomas; 1994.

APPENDICES

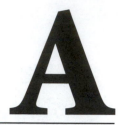

Online Clinical Teaching Resources

CLINICAL TEACHING

Kirksville College of Osteopathic Medicine Preceptor Training Resources
www.atsu.edu/kcom/preceptors/education/web_resources.htm

Clinical Teaching Perception Inventory
www.ucimc.netouch.com/index.html

Resident's Teaching Skills Website
www.ucimc.netouch.com

UC Berkeley's Office of Educational Development
teaching.berkeley.edu/compendium

Expert Preceptor Interactive Curriculum
www.med.unc.edu/epic

CLINICAL EDUCATION JOURNALS/NEWSLETTERS

Teaching and Learning in Medicine
www.siumed.edu/tlm

CLINICAL EDUCATION LIST SERVES

Athletic Training Education
http://health.groups.yahoo.com/group/athletic_training_education

Dr-Ed List Serve Archives
http://list.msu.edu/archives/dr-ed.html

CLINICAL EDUCATION PROFESSIONAL ORGANIZATIONS/COMMITTEES

NATA PEC
www.nataec.org/Committees/ProfessionalEducationCommitteePEC/tabid/58/Default.aspx

International Association of Medical Science Educators
www.iamse.org

Association of Schools of Allied Health Professions
www.asahp.org

STANDARDIZED PATIENT RESOURCES

Association of Standardized Patient Educators
www.aspeducators.org

University of Virginia School of Medicine Clinical Skills Training and Assessment Program
www.healthsystem.virginia.edu/cstap

University of Washington Health Sciences Use of Standardized Patients
http://depts.washington.edu/hsasf/clinical/standardpts.html

B

CIE Evaluation of ACI Form

I. Purpose

The purpose of this form is to help select, train, and evaluate Approved Clinical Instructors (ACI's) for athletic training. We recommend that the seven standards and associated criteria listed below be used as guidelines, not as minimal requirements. These standards/criteria were developed in a National Athletic Trainers' Association —Research and Education Foundation research project and are considered to be clear, necessary, and appropriate for ACI's in a variety of athletic training clinical education settings.

II. Identification of Clinician

Name: _____

BOC Certification #: _____

Credentialed to practice in State? (if applicable) ____ Yes ____ No

Years of clinical experience: _____

Employment setting

_____ College/University Athletic Training Facility

_____ High School Athletic Training Facility

_____ Community-Based Health Care Facility (eg, sports medicine clinic)

Date: _____

Name of institution/setting: _____

Name of person completing form: _____

Position of person completing form: _____

Address: _____

Street: _____ City: _____ State: ___ Zip: _____

Telephone: (____) _____ Email: _____

III. Definition of Terms

Approved Clinical Instructor: An Approved Clinical Instructor (ACI) is a BOC Certified Athletic Trainer with a minimum of one year of work experience as an athletic trainer, and who has completed Approved Clinical Instructor training. An ACI provides formal instruction and evaluation of clinical proficiencies in classroom, laboratory, and/or in clinical education experiences through direct supervision of athletic training students.

Clinical Instructor: A Clinical Instructor (CI) is a BOC certified athletic trainer or other qualified health care professional with a minimum of one year work experience in their respective academic or clinical area. Clinical instructors teach, evaluate, and supervise athletic training students in the field experiences. A clinical instructor is not charged with the final formal evaluation of athletic training students' integration of clinical proficiencies. A clinical instructor may also be an ACI.

IV. Use the Standards and Associated Criteria Below as Guidelines to Select, Train, and/or Evaluate an ACI

Standard 1.0

The approved clinical instructor (ACI) demonstrates legal and ethical behavior that meets the expectations of members of the profession of athletic training.

Use the following scale to respond to the criteria listed below for this standard:

1 = Never   2 = Seldom   3 = Occasionally   4 = Usually   5 = Always

Criterion 1.1

The ACI holds the appropriate credential [BOC certification and state license, registration, certification, or exemption, if applicable] as required by the state in which the individual provides athletic training services.

Yes _____   No _____

Criterion 1.2

The ACI provides athletic training services that are defined by the Role Delineation Study and within the scope of the respective state practice act (if applicable).

1   2   3   4   5   Unknown

Criterion 1.3

The ACI provides athletic training services that are consistent with state and federal legislation. Examples include equal opportunity and affirmative action policies, ADA, HIPAA, and FERPA.

1   2   3   4   5   Unknown

Criterion 1.4

The ACI demonstrates ethical behavior as defined by the NATA Code of Ethics and the BOC Standards of Professional Practice.

1   2   3   4   5   Unknown

Standard 2.0

The approved clinical instructor (ACI) demonstrates effective communication skills.

Use the following scale to respond to the criteria listed below for this standard:

1 = Never   2 = Seldom   3 = Occasionally   4 = Usually   5 = Always

Criterion 2.1

The ACI communicates with the Program Director and/or Clinical Education Coordinator regarding athletic training students' progress towards clinical education goals at regularly scheduled intervals determined by the athletic training education program.

1   2   3   4   5   Unknown

Criterion 2.2

The ACI uses appropriate forms of communication to clearly and concisely express him/her to athletic training students, both verbally and in writing.

1   2   3   4   5   Unknown

Criterion 2.3

The ACI provides appropriately timed and constructive formative and summative feedback to athletic training students.

1   2   3   4   5   Unknown

Criterion 2.4

The ACI facilitates communication with athletic training students through open-ended questions and directed problem solving.

1   2   3   4   5   Unknown

Criterion 2.5

The ACI ensures time for on-going professional discussions with the athletic training student in the clinical setting.

1   2   3   4   5   Unknown

Criterion 2.6

The ACI communicates with athletic training students in a non-confrontational and positive manner.

1   2   3   4   5   Unknown

Criterion 2.7

The ACI receives and responds to feedback from the Program Director and/or Clinical Education Coordinator, and athletic training students.

1   2   3   4   5   Unknown

Standard 3.0

The approved clinical instructor (ACI) demonstrates appropriate and professional interpersonal relationships.

Use the following scale to respond to the criteria listed below for this standard:

1 = Never   2 = Seldom   3 = Occasionally   4 = Usually   5 = Always

Criterion 3.1

The ACI forms appropriate and professional relationships with athletic training students.

1   2   3   4   5   Unknown

Criterion 3.2

The ACI models appropriate and professional interpersonal relationships when interacting with athletic training students, colleagues, patients/athletes, and administrators.

1   2   3   4   5   Unknown

Criterion 3.3

The ACI appropriately advocates for athletic training students when interacting with colleagues, patients/athletes, and administrators.

1   2   3   4   5   Unknown

Criterion 3.4

The ACI is a positive role model and/or mentor for athletic training students.

1   2   3   4   5   Unknown

Criterion 3.5

The ACI demonstrates respect for gender, racial, ethnic, religious, and individual differences when interacting with people.

1   2   3   4   5   Unknown

Criterion 3.6

The ACI has an open and approachable demeanor to athletic training students when working in the clinical setting.

1   2   3   4   5   Unknown

Standard 4.0

The approved clinical instructor (ACI) demonstrates effective instructional skills.

Use the following scale to respond to the criteria listed below for this standard:

1 = Never   2 = Seldom   3 = Occasionally   4 = Usually   5 = Always

Criterion 4.1

The ACI collaborates with the Program Director and/or Clinical Education Coordinator to plan learning experiences.

1   2   3   4   5   Unknown

Criterion 4.2

The ACI implements, facilitates, and evaluates planned learning experiences with athletic training students.

1   2   3   4   5   Unknown

Criterion 4.3

The ACI understands the athletic training students' academic curriculum, level of didactic preparation, and current level of performance, relative to the goals of the clinical education experience.

1   2   3   4   5   Unknown

Criterion 4.4

The ACI takes advantage of teachable moments during planned and unplanned learning experiences by instructing skills or content that is meaningful and immediately applicable.

1   2   3   4   5   Unknown

Criterion 4.5

The ACI employs a variety of teaching styles to meet individual athletic training students' needs.

1   2   3   4   5   Unknown

Criterion 4.6

The ACI helps athletic training student's progress towards meeting the goals and objectives of the clinical experience as assigned by the Program Director and/or Clinical Education Coordinator.

1   2   3   4   5   Unknown

Criterion 4.7

The ACI modifies learning experiences based on the athletic training students' strengths and weaknesses.

1   2   3   4   5   Unknown

Criterion 4.8

The ACI creates learning opportunities that actively engage athletic training students in the clinical setting and that promote problem-solving and critical thinking.

1   2   3   4   5   Unknown

Criterion 4.9

The ACI encourages self-directed learning activities for the athletic training students when appropriate.

1   2   3   4   5   Unknown

Criterion 4.10

The ACI performs regular self-appraisal of his/her teaching methods and effectiveness.

1   2   3   4   5   Unknown

Criterion 4.11

The ACI is enthusiastic about teaching athletic training students.

1   2   3   4   5   Unknown

Criterion 4.12

The ACI communicates complicated/detailed concepts in terms that students can understand based on their level of progression within the athletic training education program.

1   2   3   4   5   Unknown

Criterion 4.13

The ACI encourages athletic training students to engage in self-directed learning as a means of establishing life-long learning practices of inquiry and clinical problem solving.

1   2   3   4   5   Unknown

Standard 5.0

The approved clinical instructor (ACI) demonstrates effective supervisory and administrative skills when working with athletic training students.

Use the following scale to respond to the criteria listed below for this standard:

1 = Never   2 = Seldom   3 = Occasionally   4 = Usually   5 = Always

Criterion 5.1

The ACI directly supervises athletic training students during formal acquisition, practice, and evaluation of the Entry-Level Athletic Training Clinical Proficiencies.

1   2   3   4   5   Unknown

Criterion 5.2

The ACI intervenes on behalf of the athlete/patient when the athletic training student is putting the athlete/patient at risk or harm.

1   2   3   4   5   Unknown

Criterion 5.3

The ACI encourages athletic training students to arrive at clinical decisions on their own according to their level of education and clinical experience.

1   2   3   4   5   Unknown

Criterion 5.4

The ACI applies the clinical education policies, procedures, and expectations of the Athletic Training Education Program.

1   2   3   4   5   Unknown

Criterion 5.5

The ACI presents clear performance expectations to athletic training students at the beginning and throughout the learning experience.

1   2   3   4   5   Unknown

Criterion 5.6

The ACI informs athletic training students of relevant policies and procedures of the clinical setting.

1   2   3   4   5   Unknown

Criterion 5.7

The ACI provides feedback to athletic training students from information acquired from direct observation, discussion with others and from review of athlete/patient documentation.

1   2   3   4   5   Unknown

Criterion 5.8

The ACI treats the athletic training students' presence as educational and not as a means for providing medical coverage.

1   2   3   4   5   Unknown

Criterion 5.9

The ACI completes athletic training students' evaluation forms requested for the Athletic Training Education Program in a timely fashion.

1   2   3   4   5   Unknown

Criterion 5.10

The ACI provides the Program Director and/or Clinical Education Coordinator with requested materials as required for the accreditation process.

1   2   3   4   5   Unknown

Criterion 5.11

The ACI collaborates with athletic training students to arrange quality clinical education experiences that are compatible with the students' academic schedule.

1   2   3   4   5   Unknown

Standard 6.0

The approved clinical instructor (ACI) effectively evaluates athletic training student performance.

Use the following scale to respond to the criteria listed below for this standard:

1 = Never   2 = Seldom   3 = Occasionally   4 = Usually   5 = Always

Criterion 6.1

The ACI notes the athletic training students' knowledge, skills, and behaviors as they relate to the specific goals and objectives of their clinical experience.

1   2   3   4   5   Unknown

Criterion 6.2

The ACI communicates with the Program Director and/or Clinical Education Coordinator regarding implementing and/or clarifying the Athletic Training Education Program's performance evaluation instruments.

1   2   3   4   5   Unknown

Criterion 6.3

The ACI records student progress based on performance criteria established by the Athletic Training Education Program and identifies areas of competence as well as areas that require improvement.

1   2   3   4   5   Unknown

Criterion 6.4

The ACI approaches the evaluation process as constructive and educational.

1   2   3   4   5   Unknown

Criterion 6.5

The ACI communicates with the Program Director and/or Clinical Education Coordinator in a timely manner when an athletic training student needs remediation.

| 1 | 2 | 3 | 4 | 5 | Unknown |

Criterion 6.6

The ACI and athletic training students participate in formative (ie, on-going specific feedback) and summative (ie, general overall performance feedback) evaluations.

| 1 | 2 | 3 | 4 | 5 | Unknown |

Standard 7.0

The approved clinical instructor (ACI) demonstrates clinical skills and knowledge which meet or exceed the athletic training education competencies and clinical proficiencies.

Use the following scale to respond to the criteria listed below for this standard:

1 = Never   2 = Seldom   3 = Occasionally   4 = Usually   5 = Always

Criterion 7.1

The ACI is capable of teaching and evaluating the clinical proficiencies that are particular to their setting or environment.

| 1 | 2 | 3 | 4 | 5 | Unknown |

Criterion 7.2

The ACI's knowledge and skills are current and support care decisions based on science and evidence-based practice.

| 1 | 2 | 3 | 4 | 5 | Unknown |

Criterion 7.3

The ACI maintains his/her clinical skills and knowledge through participation in continuing education programs.

| 1 | 2 | 3 | 4 | 5 | Unknown |

Comments regarding strengths, weaknesses, and/or suggestions for improvement:

Funding support provided by the National Athletic Trainers' Association Research and Education Foundation, 2002

Work completed by Thomas G. Weidner, PHD, ATC/L and Jolene M. Henning, EdD, ATC-L

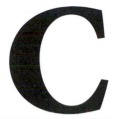

ACI Self-Evaluation Form

I. PURPOSE

The purpose of this form is to help an ACI to self-evaluate their clinical instruction. It can be used as a point of reflection on an ACI's current educational practices and therefore provide a plan of action for the modification of those practices that will lead to higher quality clinical instruction for athletic training students. We recommend that the seven standards and associated criteria listed below be used as guidelines, not as minimal requirements. These standards/criteria were developed in a National Athletic Trainers' Association—Research and Education Foundation research project and are considered to be clear, necessary, and appropriate for ACIs in a variety of athletic training clinical education settings.

II. IDENTIFICATION OF APPROVED CLINICAL INSTRUCTOR

Name: _____

Years of experience as an Approved Clinical Instructor: _____

Date: _____

Employment setting

_____ College/University Athletic Training Facility

_____ High School Athletic Training Facility

_____ Community-Based Health Care Facility (eg, sports medicine clinic)

Date: _____

Name of institution/setting: _____

Name of person completing form: _____

Position of person completing form: _____

Address: _____

Street: _____ City: _____ State: ____ Zip: _____

Telephone: (_____) _____ Email: _____

III. Definition of Terms

Approved Clinical Instructor: An Approved Clinical Instructor (ACI) is a BOC Certified Athletic Trainer with a minimum of one year of work experience as an athletic trainer, and who has completed Approved Clinical Instructor training. An ACI provides formal instruction and evaluation of clinical proficiencies in classroom, laboratory, and/or in clinical education experiences through direct supervision of athletic training students.

Clinical Instructor: A clinical instructor (CI) is a BOC certified athletic trainer or other qualified health care professional with a minimum of one year of work experience in their respective academic or clinical area. Clinical instructors teach, evaluate, and supervise athletic training students in the field experiences. A clinical instructor is not charged with the final formal evaluation of athletic training students' integration of clinical proficiencies. A clinical instructor may also be an ACI.

IV. Use the Standards and Associated Criteria Below as Guidelines to Self-Evaluate Your Performance as an ACI

Standard 1.0

The approved clinical instructor (ACI) demonstrates legal and ethical behavior that meets the expectations of members of the profession of athletic training.

Use the following scale to respond to the criteria listed below for this standard:

1 = Never   2 = Seldom   3 = Occasionally   4 = Usually   5 = Always

Criterion 1.1

As an ACI, I hold the appropriate credential [BOC certification and state license, registration, certification, or exemption, if applicable] as required by the state in which I provide athletic training services.

Yes ＿＿   No ＿＿   Unknown ＿＿

Criterion 1.2

As an ACI, I provide athletic training services that are defined by the Role Delineation Study and within the scope of the respective state practice act (if applicable).

1   2   3   4   5   Unknown

Criterion 1.3

As an ACI, I provide athletic training services that are consistent with state and federal legislation. Examples include equal opportunity and affirmative action policies, ADA, HIPAA, and FERPA.

1   2   3   4   5   Unknown

Criterion 1.4

As an ACI, I demonstrate ethical behavior as defined by the NATA Code of Ethics and the BOC Standards of Professional Practice.

1   2   3   4   5   Unknown

Standard 2.0

The approved clinical instructor (ACI) demonstrates effective communication skills.

Use the following scale to respond to the criteria listed below for this standard:

1 = Never   2 = Seldom   3 = Occasionally   4 = Usually   5 = Always

Criterion 2.1

As an ACI, I communicate with the Program Director and/or Clinical Education Coordinator regarding athletic training student progress towards clinical education goals at regularly scheduled intervals determined by the athletic training education program.

1   2   3   4   5   Unknown

Criterion 2.2

As an ACI, I use appropriate forms of communication to clearly and concisely express myself to athletic training students, both verbally and in writing.

1   2   3   4   5   Unknown

Criterion 2.3

As an ACI, I provide appropriately timed and constructive formative and summative feedback to athletic training students.

1   2   3   4   5   Unknown

Criterion 2.4

As an ACI, I facilitate communication with athletic training students through open-ended questions and directed problem solving.

1   2   3   4   5   Unknown

Criterion 2.5

As an ACI, I ensure time for on-going professional discussions with the athletic training student in the clinical setting.

1   2   3   4   5   Unknown

Criterion 2.6

As an ACI, I communicate with athletic training students in a non-confrontational and positive manner.

1   2   3   4   5   Unknown

Criterion 2.7

As an ACI, I receive and respond to, feedback from the Program Director and/or Clinical Education Coordinator, and athletic training students.

| 1 | 2 | 3 | 4 | 5 | Unknown |

Standard 3.0

The approved clinical instructor (ACI) demonstrates appropriate and professional interpersonal relationships.

Use the following scale to respond to the criteria listed below for this standard:

1 = Never   2 = Seldom   3 = Occasionally   4 = Usually   5 = Always

Criterion 3.1

As an ACI, I form appropriate and professional relationships with athletic training students.

| 1 | 2 | 3 | 4 | 5 | Unknown |

Criterion 3.2

As an ACI, I model appropriate and professional interpersonal relationships when interacting with athletic training students, colleagues, patients/athletes, and administrators.

| 1 | 2 | 3 | 4 | 5 | Unknown |

Criterion 3.3

As an ACI, I appropriately advocate athletic training students when interacting with colleagues, patients/athletes, and administrators.

| 1 | 2 | 3 | 4 | 5 | Unknown |

Criterion 3.4

As an ACI, I am a positive role model and/or mentor for athletic training students.

| 1 | 2 | 3 | 4 | 5 | Unknown |

Criterion 3.5

As an ACI, I demonstrate respect for gender, racial, ethnic, religious, and individual differences when interacting with people.

| 1 | 2 | 3 | 4 | 5 | Unknown |

Criterion 3.6

As an ACI, I have an open and approachable demeanor to athletic training students when working in the clinical setting.

| 1 | 2 | 3 | 4 | 5 | Unknown |

Standard 4.0

The approved clinical instructor (ACI) demonstrates effective instructional skills.

Use the following scale to respond to the criteria listed below for this standard:

1 = Never   2 = Seldom   3 = Occasionally   4 = Usually   5 = Always

Criterion 4.1

As an ACI, I collaborate with the Program Director and/or Clinical Education Coordinator to plan learning experiences.

| 1 | 2 | 3 | 4 | 5 | Unknown |

Criterion 4.2

As an ACI, I implement, facilitate, and evaluate planned learning experiences with athletic training students.

| 1 | 2 | 3 | 4 | 5 | Unknown |

Criterion 4.3

As an ACI, I understand the athletic training students' academic curriculum, level of didactic preparation, and current level of performance, relative to the goals of the clinical education experience.

| 1 | 2 | 3 | 4 | 5 | Unknown |

Criterion 4.4

As an ACI, I take advantage of teachable moments during planned and unplanned learning experiences by instructing skills or content that is meaningful and immediately applicable.

| 1 | 2 | 3 | 4 | 5 | Unknown |

Criterion 4.5

As an ACI, I employ a variety of teaching styles to meet individual athletic training students' needs.

| 1 | 2 | 3 | 4 | 5 | Unknown |

Criterion 4.6

As an ACI, I help athletic training student's progress towards meeting the goals and objectives of the clinical experience as assigned by the Program Director and/or Clinical Education Coordinator.

| 1 | 2 | 3 | 4 | 5 | Unknown |

Criterion 4.7

As an ACI, I modify learning experiences based on the athletic training students' strengths and weaknesses.

| 1 | 2 | 3 | 4 | 5 | Unknown |

Criterion 4.8

As an ACI, I create learning opportunities that actively engage athletic training students in the clinical setting and that promote problem-solving and critical thinking.

| 1 | 2 | 3 | 4 | 5 | Unknown |

Criterion 4.9

As an ACI, I encourage self-directed learning activities for the athletic training students when appropriate.

| 1 | 2 | 3 | 4 | 5 | Unknown |

Criterion 4.10

As an ACI, I perform regular self-appraisal of my teaching methods and effectiveness.

| 1 | 2 | 3 | 4 | 5 | Unknown |

Criterion 4.11

As an ACI, I am enthusiastic about teaching athletic training students.

| 1 | 2 | 3 | 4 | 5 | Unknown |

Criterion 4.12

As an ACI, I communicate complicated/detailed concepts in terms that students can understand based on their level of progression within the athletic training education program.

| 1 | 2 | 3 | 4 | 5 | Unknown |

Criterion 4.13

As an ACI, I encourage athletic training students to engage in self-directed learning as a means of establishing life-long learning practices of inquiry and clinical problem solving.

| 1 | 2 | 3 | 4 | 5 | Unknown |

Standard 5.0

The approved clinical instructor (ACI) demonstrates effective supervisory and administrative skills when working with athletic training students.

Use the following scale to respond to the criteria listed below for this standard:

1 = Never   2 = Seldom   3 = Occasionally   4 = Usually   5 = Always

Criterion 5.1

As an ACI, I directly supervise athletic training students during formal acquisition, practice, and evaluation of the Entry-Level Athletic Training Clinical Proficiencies.

| 1 | 2 | 3 | 4 | 5 | Unknown |

Criterion 5.2

As an ACI, I intervene on behalf of the athlete/patient when the athletic training student is putting the athlete/patient at risk or harm.

1   2   3   4   5   Unknown

Criterion 5.3

As an ACI, I encourage athletic training students to arrive at clinical decisions on their own according to their level of education and clinical experience.

1   2   3   4   5   Unknown

Criterion 5.4

As an ACI, I apply the clinical education policies, procedures, and expectations of the Athletic Training Education Program.

1   2   3   4   5   Unknown

Criterion 5.5

As an ACI, I present clear performance expectations to athletic training students at the beginning and throughout the learning experience.

1   2   3   4   5   Unknown

Criterion 5.6

As an ACI, I inform athletic training students of relevant policies and procedures of the clinical setting.

1   2   3   4   5   Unknown

Criterion 5.7

As an ACI, I provide feedback to athletic training students from information acquired from direct observation, discussion with others and from review of athlete/patient documentation.

1   2   3   4   5   Unknown

Criterion 5.8

As an ACI, I treat the athletic training students' presence as educational and not as a means for providing medical coverage.

1   2   3   4   5   Unknown

Criterion 5.9

As an ACI, I complete athletic training students' evaluation forms requested for the Athletic Training Education Program in a timely fashion.

1   2   3   4   5   Unknown

Criterion 5.10

As an ACI, I provide the Program Director and/or Clinical Education Coordinator with requested materials as required for the accreditation process.

1   2   3   4   5   Unknown

Criterion 5.11

As an ACI, I collaborate with athletic training students to arrange quality clinical education experiences which are compatible with the students' academic schedule.

1   2   3   4   5   Unknown

Standard 6.0

The approved clinical instructor (ACI) effectively evaluates athletic training student performance.

Use the following scale to respond to the criteria listed below for this standard:

1 = Never   2 = Seldom   3 = Occasionally   4 = Usually   5 = Always

Criterion 6.1

As an ACI, I note the athletic training students' knowledge, skills, and behaviors as they relate to the specific goals and objectives of their clinical experience.

1   2   3   4   5   Unknown

Criterion 6.2

As an ACI, I communicate with the Program Director and/or Clinical Education Coordinator regarding implementing and/or clarifying the Athletic Training Education Program's performance evaluation instruments.

1   2   3   4   5   Unknown

Criterion 6.3

As an ACI, I record student progress based on performance criteria established by the Athletic Training Education Program and identifies areas of competence as well as areas that require improvement.

1   2   3   4   5   Unknown

Criterion 6.4

As an ACI, I approach the evaluation process as constructive and educational.

1   2   3   4   5   Unknown

Criterion 6.5

As an ACI, I communicate with the Program Director and/or Clinical Education Coordinator in a timely manner when an athletic training student needs remediation.

1   2   3   4   5   Unknown

Criterion 6.6

As an ACI, I and the athletic training students participate in formative (ie, on-going specific feedback) and summative (ie, general overall performance feedback) evaluations.

| 1 | 2 | 3 | 4 | 5 | Unknown |

Standard 7.0

The approved clinical instructor (ACI) demonstrates clinical skills and knowledge which meet or exceed the athletic training education competencies and clinical proficiencies.

Use the following scale to respond to the criteria listed below for this standard:

1 = Never   2 = Seldom   3 = Occasionally   4 = Usually   5 = Always

Criterion 7.1

As an ACI, I am capable of teaching and evaluating the clinical proficiencies which are particular to their setting or environment.

| 1 | 2 | 3 | 4 | 5 | Unknown |

Criterion 7.2

As an ACI, my knowledge and skills are current and support care decisions based on science and evidence-based practice.

| 1 | 2 | 3 | 4 | 5 | Unknown |

Criterion 7.3

As an ACI, I maintain my clinical skills and knowledge through participation in continuing education programs.

| 1 | 2 | 3 | 4 | 5 | Unknown |

Comments regarding strengths, weaknesses, and/or suggestions for improvement:

Funding support provided by the National Athletic Trainers' Association Research and Education Foundation, 2002

Work completed by Thomas G. Weidner, PhD, ATC/L and Jolene M. Henning, EdD, ATC-L

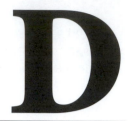

Student/Peer Evaluation of ACI Form

I. Purpose

The purpose of this form is to help athletic training students and clinical instructor colleagues to evaluate the clinical instruction of an ACI. We recommend that the seven standards and associated criteria listed below be used as guidelines, not as minimal requirements. These standards/criteria were developed in a National Athletic Trainers' Association - Research and Education Foundation research project and are considered to be clear, necessary, and appropriate for ACI's in a variety of athletic training clinical education settings.

II. Identification of Approved Clinical Instructor

Name of ACI: _____

Please check if you are: Colleague _____   or   Student _____

Date: _____

Employment setting

_____ College/University Athletic Training Facility

_____ High School Athletic Training Facility

_____ Community-Based Health Care Facility (eg, sports medicine clinic)

Name of institution/setting: _____

Name of person completing form: _____

Position of person completing form: _____

Address: _____

Street: _____ City: _____ State: ____ Zip: _____

Telephone: (_____) _____ Email: _____

III. DEFINITION OF TERMS

Approved Clinical Instructor: An Approved Clinical Instructor (ACI) is a BOC Certified Athletic Trainer with a minimum of one year of work experience as an athletic trainer, and who has completed Approved Clinical Instructor training. An ACI provides formal instruction and evaluation of clinical proficiencies in classroom, laboratory, and/or in clinical education experiences through direct supervision of athletic training students.

Clinical Instructor: A clinical instructor (CI) is a BOC certified athletic trainer or other qualified health care professional with a minimum of one year of work experience in their respective academic or clinical area. Clinical instructors teach, evaluate, and supervise athletic training students in the field experiences. A clinical instructor is not charged with the final formal evaluation of athletic training students' integration of clinical proficiencies. A clinical instructor may also be an ACI.

IV. USE THE STANDARDS AND ASSOCIATED CRITERIA BELOW AS GUIDELINES TO EVALUATE THE PERFORMANCE OF AN ACI

Standard 1.0

The approved clinical instructor (ACI) demonstrates legal and ethical behavior that meets the expectations of members of the profession of athletic training.

Use the following scale to respond to the criteria listed below for this standard:

1 = Never   2 = Seldom   3 = Occasionally   4 = Usually   5 = Always

Criterion 1.1

The ACI holds the appropriate credential [BOC certification and state license, registration, certification, or exemption, if applicable] as required by the state in which the individual provides athletic training services.

Yes ____   No _____   Unknown _____

Criterion 1.2

The ACI provides athletic training services that are defined by the Role Delineation Study and within the scope of the respective state practice act (if applicable).

1   2   3   4   5   Unknown

Criterion 1.3

The ACI provides athletic training services that are consistent with state and federal legislation. Examples include equal opportunity and affirmative action policies, ADA, HIPAA, and FERPA.

1   2   3   4   5   Unknown

Criterion 1.4

The ACI demonstrates ethical behavior as defined by the NATA Code of Ethics and the BOC Standards of Professional Practice.

1   2   3   4   5   Unknown

Standard 2.0

The approved clinical instructor (ACI) demonstrates effective communication skills.

Use the following scale to respond to the criteria listed below for this standard:

1 = Never   2 = Seldom   3 = Occasionally   4 = Usually   5 = Always

Criterion 2.1

The ACI communicates with the Program Director and/or Clinical Education Coordinator regarding athletic training student progress towards clinical education goals at regularly scheduled intervals determined by the athletic training education program.

1   2   3   4   5   Unknown

Criterion 2.2

The ACI uses appropriate forms of communication to clearly and concisely express him/her to athletic training students, both verbally and in writing.

1   2   3   4   5   Unknown

Criterion 2.3

The ACI provides appropriately timed and constructive formative and summative feedback to athletic training students.

1   2   3   4   5   Unknown

Criterion 2.4

The ACI facilitates communication with athletic training students through open-ended questions and directed problem solving.

1   2   3   4   5   Unknown

Criterion 2.5

The ACI ensures time for on-going professional discussions with the athletic training student in the clinical setting.

1   2   3   4   5   Unknown

Criterion 2.6

The ACI communicates with athletic training students in a nonconfrontational and positive manner.

1   2   3   4   5   Unknown

Criterion 2.7

The ACI receives and responds to, feedback from the Program Director and/or Clinical Education Coordinator, and athletic training students.

1   2   3   4   5   Unknown

Standard 3.0

The approved clinical instructor (ACI) demonstrates appropriate and professional interpersonal relationships.

Use the following scale to respond to the criteria listed below for this standard:

1 = Never   2 = Seldom   3 = Occasionally   4 = Usually   5 = Always

Criterion 3.1

The ACI forms appropriate and professional relationships with athletic training students.

1   2   3   4   5   Unknown

Criterion 3.2

The ACI models appropriate and professional interpersonal relationships when interacting with athletic training students, colleagues, patients/athletes, and administrators.

1   2   3   4   5   Unknown

Criterion 3.3

The ACI appropriately advocates athletic training students when interacting with colleagues, patients/athletes, and administrators.

1   2   3   4   5   Unknown

Criterion 3.4

The ACI is a positive role model and/or mentor for athletic training students.

1   2   3   4   5   Unknown

Criterion 3.5

The ACI demonstrates respect for gender, racial, ethnic, religious, and individual differences when interacting with people.

1   2   3   4   5   Unknown

Criterion 3.6

The ACI has an open and approachable demeanor to athletic training students when working in the clinical setting.

1   2   3   4   5   Unknown

Standard 4.0

The approved clinical instructor (ACI) demonstrates effective instructional skills.

Use the following scale to respond to the criteria listed below for this standard:

1 = Never   2 = Seldom   3 = Occasionally   4 = Usually   5 = Always

Criterion 4.1

The ACI collaborates with the Program Director and/or Clinical Education Coordinator to plan learning experiences.

1   2   3   4   5   Unknown

Criterion 4.2

The ACI implements, facilitates, and evaluates planned learning experiences with athletic training students.

1   2   3   4   5   Unknown

Criterion 4.3

The ACI understands the athletic training students' academic curriculum, level of didactic preparation, and current level of performance, relative to the goals of the clinical education experience.

1   2   3   4   5   Unknown

Criterion 4.4

The ACI takes advantage of teachable moments during planned and unplanned learning experiences by instructing skills or content that is meaningful and immediately applicable.

1   2   3   4   5   Unknown

Criterion 4.5

The ACI employs a variety of teaching styles to meet individual athletic training students' needs.

1   2   3   4   5   Unknown

Criterion 4.6

The ACI helps athletic training student's progress towards meeting the goals and objectives of the clinical experience as assigned by the Program Director and/or Clinical Education Coordinator.

1   2   3   4   5   Unknown

Criterion 4.7

The ACI modifies learning experiences based on the athletic training students' strengths and weaknesses.

1   2   3   4   5   Unknown

Criterion 4.8

The ACI creates learning opportunities that actively engage athletic training students in the clinical setting and that promote problem-solving and critical thinking.

1   2   3   4   5   Unknown

Criterion 4.9

The ACI encourages self-directed learning activities for the athletic training students when appropriate.

1   2   3   4   5   Unknown

Criterion 4.10

The ACI performs regular self-appraisal of his/her teaching methods and effectiveness.

1   2   3   4   5   Unknown

Criterion 4.11

The ACI is enthusiastic about teaching athletic training students.

1   2   3   4   5   Unknown

Criterion 4.12

The ACI communicates complicated/detailed concepts in terms that students can understand based on their level of progression within the athletic training education program.

1   2   3   4   5   Unknown

Criterion 4.13

The ACI encourages athletic training students to engage in self-directed learning as a means of establishing life-long learning practices of inquiry and clinical problem solving.

1   2   3   4   5   Unknown

Standard 5.0

The approved clinical instructor (ACI) demonstrates effective supervisory and administrative skills when working with athletic training students.

Use the following scale to respond to the criteria listed below for this standard:

1 = Never   2 = Seldom   3 = Occasionally   4 = Usually   5 = Always

Criterion 5.1

The ACI directly supervises athletic training students during formal acquisition, practice, and evaluation of the Entry-Level Athletic Training Clinical Proficiencies.

1   2   3   4   5   Unknown

Criterion 5.2

The ACI intervenes on behalf of the athlete/patient when the athletic training student is putting the athlete/patient at risk or harm.

1   2   3   4   5   Unknown

Criterion 5.3

The ACI encourages athletic training students to arrive at clinical decisions on their own according to their level of education and clinical experience.

1   2   3   4   5   Unknown

Criterion 5.4

The ACI applies the clinical education policies, procedures, and expectations of the Athletic Training Education Program.

1   2   3   4   5   Unknown

Criterion 5.5

The ACI presents clear performance expectations to athletic training students at the beginning and throughout the learning experience.

1   2   3   4   5   Unknown

Criterion 5.6

The ACI informs athletic training students of relevant policies and procedures of the clinical setting.

1   2   3   4   5   Unknown

Criterion 5.7

The ACI provides feedback to athletic training students from information acquired from direct observation, discussion with others and from review of athlete/patient documentation.

1   2   3   4   5   Unknown

Criterion 5.8

The ACI treats the athletic training students' presence as educational and not as a means for providing medical coverage.

1   2   3   4   5   Unknown

Criterion 5.9

The ACI completes athletic training students' evaluation forms requested for the Athletic Training Education Program in a timely fashion.

1   2   3   4   5   Unknown

Criterion 5.10

The ACI provides the Program Director and/or Clinical Education Coordinator with requested materials as required for the accreditation process.

1   2   3   4   5   Unknown

Criterion 5.11

The ACI collaborates with athletic training students to arrange quality clinical education experiences which are compatible with the students' academic schedule.

1   2   3   4   5   Unknown

Standard 6.0

The approved clinical instructor (ACI) effectively evaluates athletic training student performance.

Use the following scale to respond to the criteria listed below for this standard:

1 = Never   2 = Seldom   3 = Occasionally   4 = Usually   5 = Always

Criterion 6.1

The ACI notes the athletic training students' knowledge, skills, and behaviors as they relate to the specific goals and objectives of their clinical experience.

1   2   3   4   5   Unknown

Criterion 6.2

The ACI communicates with the Program Director and/or Clinical Education Coordinator regarding implementing and/or clarifying the Athletic Training Education Program's performance evaluation instruments.

1   2   3   4   5   Unknown

Criterion 6.3

The ACI records student progress based on performance criteria established by the Athletic Training Education Program and identifies areas of competence as well as areas that require improvement.

1   2   3   4   5   Unknown

Criterion 6.4

The ACI approaches the evaluation process as constructive and educational.

1   2   3   4   5   Unknown

Criterion 6.5

The ACI communicates with the Program Director and/or Clinical Education Coordinator in a timely manner when an athletic training student needs remediation.

1   2   3   4   5   Unknown

Criterion 6.6

The ACI and athletic training students participate in formative (ie, on-going specific feedback) and summative (ie, general overall performance feedback) evaluations.

1   2   3   4   5   Unknown

Standard 7.0

The approved clinical instructor (ACI) demonstrates clinical skills and knowledge that meet or exceed the athletic training education competencies and clinical proficiencies.

Use the following scale to respond to the criteria listed below for this standard:

1 = Never   2 = Seldom   3 = Occasionally   4 = Usually   5 = Always

Criterion 7.1

The ACI is capable of teaching and evaluating the clinical proficiencies that are particular to their setting or environment.

1   2   3   4   5   Unknown

Criterion 7.2

The ACI's knowledge and skills are current and support care decisions based on science and evidence-based practice.

1   2   3   4   5   Unknown

Criterion 7.3

The ACI maintains his/her clinical skills and knowledge through participation in continuing education programs.

1   2   3   4   5   Unknown

Comments regarding strengths, weaknesses, and/or suggestions for improvement:

Funding support provided by the National Athletic Trainers' Association Research and Education Foundation, 2002

Work completed by Thomas G. Weidner, PhD, ATC/L and Jolene M. Henning, EdD, ATC-L

Foundational Behaviors of Professional Practice

These basic behaviors permeate every aspect of professional practice, and should be incorporated into instruction in every part of the educational program. The behaviors in this section comprise the application of the common values of the athletic training profession.

PRIMACY OF THE PATIENT

- Recognize sources of conflict of interest that can impact the patient's health
- Know and apply the commonly accepted standards for patient confidentiality
- Provide the best health care available for the patient
- Advocate for the needs of the patient

TEAMED APPROACH TO PRACTICE

- Recognize the unique skills and abilities of other health care professionals
- Understand the scope of practice of other health care professionals
- Understand and execute duties within the identified scope of practice for athletic trainers
- Include the patient (and family, where appropriate) in the decision making process
- Demonstrate the ability to work with others in effecting positive patient outcomes

LEGAL PRACTICE

- Practice athletic training in a legally competent manner
- Recognize the need to document compliance with the laws that govern athletic training

- Understand the consequences of violating the laws that govern athletic training

ETHICAL PRACTICE

- Understand and comply with the NATA's Code of Ethics and the BOC's Standards of Practice
- Understand the consequences of violating the NATA's Code of Ethics and BOC's Standards of Practice
- Understand and comply with other codes of ethics, as applicable.

ADVANCING KNOWLEDGE

- Critically examine the body of knowledge in athletic training and related fields
- Use evidence-based practice as a foundation for the delivery of care
- Understand the connection between continuing education and the improvement of athletic training practice
- Promote the value of research and scholarship in athletic training
- Disseminate new knowledge in athletic training to fellow athletic trainers, patients, other health care professionals, and others as necessary

CULTURAL COMPETENCE

- Understand the cultural differences of patients' attitudes and behaviors toward health care
- Demonstrate knowledge, attitudes, behaviors, and skills necessary to achieve optimal health outcomes for diverse patient populations.
- Demonstrate knowledge, attitudes, behaviors, and skills necessary to work respectfully and effectively with diverse populations and in a diverse work environment

PROFESSIONALISM

- Advocate for the profession
- Demonstrate honesty and integrity
- Exhibit compassion and empathy
- Demonstrate effective interpersonal communication skills

National Athletic Trainers' Association. *Athletic Training Educational Competencies*. 4th ed. Dallas, TX: National Athletic Trainers' Association; 2006.

Clinical Education Setting Student Assessment Form

1. Level in ATEP
   a. Beginning student (1st or 2nd semester)
   b. Intermediate student (3rd or 4th semester)
   c. Advanced student (5th or 6th semester)

2. Clinical setting name

3. Clinical setting type
   a. College/university athletic training facility
   b. High school athletic training facility
   c. Community-based health care facility (eg, sports medicine clinic)

DIRECTIONS:

Please evaluate the Clinical Education Setting for athletic training. Please check the appropriate response in each category. If a response does not apply, please select the NA option.

Please indicate the helpfulness of the opportunities made available to you prior to your clinical education experience

SECTION I: ORIENTATION

4. Patients/athletes served
   a. Not available/not helpful
   b. Not available/would be helpful
   c. Available/little help
   d. NA

5. Rules, regulations, & procedures
   a. Not available/not helpful
   b. Not available/would be helpful
   c. Available/little help
   d. NA

6. Objectives
   a. Not available/not helpful
   b. Not available/would be helpful
   c. Available/little help
   d. NA

7. Schedule
   a. Not available/not helpful
   b. Not available/would be helpful
   c. Available/little help
   d. NA

8. Dress code
   a. Not available/not helpful
   b. Not available/would be helpful
   c. Available/little help
   d. NA

9. Time required
   a. Not available/not helpful
   b. Not available/would be helpful
   c. Available/little help
   d. NA

10. Clinical setting objectives
    a. Not available/not helpful
    b. Not available/would be helpful
    c. Available/little help
    d. NA

11. Ethical standards of practice
    a. Not available/not helpful
    b. Not available/would be helpful
    c. Available/little help
    d. NA

12. Organization Chart
    a. Not available/not helpful
    b. Not available/would be helpful
    c. Available/little help
    d. NA

13. Were you given adequate orientation to individual patients/athletes and to your responsibilities to these people?
    a. Yes
    b. No

14. Did you have a clear understanding of what was expected of you?
    a. Yes
    b. No

15. Were your objectives for clinical education considered in planning your learning experience?
    a. Yes
    b. No

16. Did you feel that the learning experiences at this setting were?
    a. Routine for every student
    b. Individualized for every student

17. Were on-going changes made in your learning experiences based on the level of competency you demonstrated?
    a. Yes
    b. No

18. Were you provided with adequate space to accommodate your professional and personal needs (eg, lockers, study space, treatment areas)?
    a. Yes
    b. No

SECTION II: INTERACTIONS

19. Radiology technicians
    a. Yes
    b. No
    c. NA

20. Nurses
     a. Yes
     b. No
     c. NA

21. Occupational therapists
     a. Yes
     b. No
     c. NA

22. Orthotists
     a. Yes
     b. No
     c. NA

23. Paramedics/EMT's
     a. Yes
     b. No
     c. NA

24. Physical therapists
     a. Yes
     b. No
     c. NA

25. Orthopedists
     a. Yes
     b. No
     c. NA

26. Physicians
     a. Yes
     b. No
     c. NA

27. Physician's assistants
     a. Yes
     b. No
     c. NA

28. Chiropractors
    a. Yes
    b. No
    c. NA

SECTION III: IMPRESSIONS

29. Please identify other physicians not listed that you had the opportunity to interact with:

30. Please identify other health professionals not listed that you had the opportunity to interact with:

31. Did you have adequate individual attention?
    a. Yes
    b. No

32. How would you describe your patient/athlete load during the majority of your clinical education experience?
    a. Appropriate for your educational level
    b. Too high
    c. Too low

33. Please comment if you felt the patient/athlete load was too high or too low:

34. Were the variety of patients/athletes adequate to meet the objectives of the clinical education experience?
    a. Yes
    b. No

35. Please comment if you felt the variety of the patient/athlete load was not adequate to meet the objectives:

36. Were the equipment and supplies adequate to meet the objectives of the clinical education experience?
    a. Yes
    b. No

37. Please comment if you felt the equipment and supplies were not adequate to meet the objectives:

38. Did the athletic training Clinical Instructors (CIs) understand your education level and education needs?
    a. Yes
    b. No

39. Did the non-athletic training Clinical Instructors (CIs) understand your education level and needs?
    a. Yes
    b. No

40. Did you have adequate opportunity for communication with the Clinical Instructor (CI) to whom you were responsible?
    a. Yes
    b. No

41. Please describe your opportunities for discussion with your Clinical Instructor (CI) by checking all appropriate responses:
    a. Daily
    b. Once per week
    c. Impromptu
    d. Midway
    e. Whenever necessary
    f. Whenever requested
    g. Final
    h. Seldom
    i. Never
    j. Had to be scheduled in advance

42. How frequently did you receive feedback on your clinical performance?
    a. Daily
    b. Midway
    c. Final

43. Based on your experiences and skill, how would you describe the degree of supervision you received?
    a. Too close
    b. Commensurate with need
    c. Not close enough

44. If the degree of supervision was not commensurate with your needs, please comment:

45. How would you describe the final evaluation process of your performance?
    a. Discussed with you prior to and after being finalized in writing.
    b. Discussed with you only prior to being finalized in writing.
    c. Discussed with you only after being finalized in writing.
    d. Not discussed

46. How would you rate staff morale?
    a. Always high
    b. Usually high
    c. Occasionally high/occasionally low
    d. Usually low

47. Was the person who was directly responsible to you adequately prepared to answer your questions?
    a. Yes
    b. No

48. Was the person directly responsible to you interested in your learning?
    a. Yes
    b. No

49. Based on your past experience in clinical education, and your concept of the "ideal" clinical education setting, how would you rate this clinical education setting?
    a. A very negative experience
    b. A waste of time
    c. Time well spent
    d. A very positive experience

50. Identify any new subject matter that you were exposed to during this clinical education experience and indicate if it should be included in the athletic training educational program.

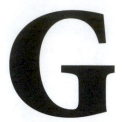

Rubric for Recognizing and Correcting Key Clinical Setting Deficiencies

Purpose: This clinical education setting assessment rubric is designed to provide you with an important opportunity to reflect on the clinical experiences that your students have reported that they received in your setting. It will help you to identify strengths and to discern areas for improvement. It is our hope that you will continue to develop and improve athletic training clinical education experiences in your setting.

Instructions: Based on your review of the Clinical Setting Evaluations that students have provided for your setting, complete (using Microsoft Word) the following self-assessment rubric. It should take approximately 15-20 minutes to complete.

Name:

Title/Position:

Name/Type of Clinical Setting:

Review your student Clinical Setting Evaluations. In addition to a numeric rating for each of the four sections, please comment on strengths and steps you can take in the next year to improve each of these sections. Use the following rating scale for this assessment:

1. Poor
2. Fair
3. Good
4. Excellent

NA Not Applicable

  I. Student Orientation to Clinical Setting:
- Strengths:
- Steps for Improvement:

II. Interactions With Other Allied Health Professionals:

- o Strengths:
- o Steps for Improvement:

III. Interactions With Patients:

- o Strengths:
- o Steps for Improvement:

IV. Interactions With Clinical Instructor(s):

- o Strengths:
- o Steps for Improvement:

Additional Comments:

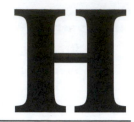

Sample Online Clinical Experience Update Report

Practicum Student's Name:

Practicum Student's E-Mail Address:

Clinical Instructor:

Practicum Site:

Rotation: 1st   2nd

Report Number: 1   2   3   4

Total Clinical Experience Hours for past 2 weeks:

DIRECTIONS

Reflect on your clinical experiences over the time period from the previous report to now. To the extent possible, it is your responsibility to make certain that you complete clinical experiences so that entries are made for each of the areas listed.

Describe your experiences regarding the following areas:

- Accepting and appreciating the roles of allied health professionals.
- Providing education and guidance on preventative techniques specific to the patient population.
- Demonstrating injury evaluation and management skills for injuries/illnesses specific to the patient population.
- Utilizing proper treatment, rehabilitation, reconditioning techniques for the injury/illness/condition specific to the patient population.
- Demonstrating an understanding of the organization and administration of sports medicine care delivered in the rehabilitation clinic and high school settings.
- Demonstrating effective communication skills with patients and allied health professionals.
- Demonstrating an appreciation of diversity and age-group characteristics of the patient population served.

- Using clinical outcome assessments through clinician-based (eg, strength, ROM) or patient-based (eg, satisfaction, return to function) measures.
- Additional comments (eg, personal appearance, dependability on completing tasks, quality of work).

CLINICAL PROFICIENCIES

- List and comment on approved clinical proficiencies that you completed during the past 2 weeks (must indicate name of ACI).
- Comment on clinical proficiencies you failed or others which you practiced during the past 2 weeks.
- Describe any evidence based medicine literature/information that you and/or your CI used or discussed during your clinical experiences.

GENERAL REMARKS

- Include any general remarks or comments in the area, below.
- This report will automatically be forwarded to your clinical and lab instructors.
- If you do not want your update report forwarded, please justify why in the box provided.
- In case of transmittal difficulty, save the confirmation report you will receive after you submit this form.

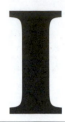

Sample Online Midterm ACI Evaluation of Student

Therapeutic Exercise/ Rehabilitation Clinic Rotation

Clinical Instructor's Name:

Student's Name:

Rotation: 1st 2nd

DIRECTIONS:

Please evaluate your student based on his/her Academic status in the Athletic Training Education Program. Note: Intermediate students (junior- level) have completed upper and lower extremity evaluation courses, and are currently enrolled in therapeutic modalities (fall semester) and therapeutic exercise (spring semester). Advanced students (senior-level) have completed these same courses and are enrolled in General Medical Conditions (fall semester).

Work Attitude: (choose one)

____ Outstanding enthusiasm

____ Very interested and industrious

____ Average in diligence and interest

____ Somewhat indifferent

Judgment: (choose one)

____ Exceptionally mature

____ Above average in making decisions

____ Usually makes the right decisions

____ Often uses poor judgment

____ Constantly uses poor judgment

Dependability in Completing Tasks: (choose one)

____ Completely dependable

____ Usually dependable

____ Sometimes neglectful or careless

____ Unreliable

Ability to Learn: (choose one)

____ Learns very quickly

____ Learns fairly quickly

____ Average in learning

____ Rather slow in learning

____ Very slow in learning

Quality of Work: (choose one)

____ Excellent

____ Very good

____ Average

____ Below average

____ Very poor

Attendance: (choose one)

____ Regular

____ Irregular

Punctuality: (choose one)

____ Regular

____ Irregular

INTERPERSONAL SKILLS

ATS demonstrates appropriate communication skills:

Verbal	1	2	3	4	5	NA
Written	1	2	3	4	5	NA
Nonverbal (body language/personal space)	1	2	3	4	5	NA

ATS demonstrates an appropriate level of empathy with injured patients/athletes.	1	2	3	4	5	NA
ATS is polite in their daily interactions with supervisors, peers, and patients.	1	2	3	4	5	NA
ATS maintains appropriate boundaries between personal and clinical experience issues.	1	2	3	4	5	NA
Critical Thinking/Problem Solving	1	2	3	4	5	NA
ATS raises relevant questions with their clinical supervisor.	1	2	3	4	5	NA
ATS raises questions at an appropriate time.	1	2	3	4	5	NA
ATS is able to recognize problems when they present.	1	2	3	4	5	NA
Treats patients/athletes without favoritism or discrimination.	1	2	3	4	5	NA

TECHNICAL STANDARDS

Mental capacity to assimilate, analyze, synthesize, integrate concepts and problem solve.	1	2	3	4	5	NA
Sufficient postural and neuromuscular control, sensory function, and coordination to perform appropriate physical examinations.	1	2	3	4	5	NA
Ability to communicate effectively and sensitively with patients and colleagues.	1	2	3	4	5	NA
Ability to record the physical examination results and a treatment plan clearly and accurately.	1	2	3	4	5	NA
Capacity to maintain composure and continue to function well during periods of high stress.	1	2	3	4	5	NA

Perseverance, diligence and commitment to complete the athletic training education program.　1　2　3　4　5　NA

Flexibility and the ability to adjust to changing situations and uncertainty in clinical situations.　1　2　3　4　5　NA

Affective skills and appropriate demeanor and rapport that relate to professional education and quality patient care.　1　2　3　4　5　NA

APPLICATION OF THERAPEUTIC EXERCISES AND TECHNIQUES

Presents methods for objectively measuring joint range of motion and their normative values for these measurements.　1　2　3　4　5　NA

Demonstrates the use of isokinetic, isotonic, and isometric exercises in the rehabilitation of injuries.　1　2　3　4　5　NA

Applies contemporary use of manual exercises in the rehabilitation of injuries.　1　2　3　4　5　NA

Designs a comprehensive rehabilitation program for an injured athlete from the point of injury to full participation.　1　2　3　4　5　NA

Designs therapeutic goals and objectives in a comprehensive rehabilitative program.　1　2　3　4　5　NA

Selects the appropriate therapeutic technique and develop criteria for progression of exercises in a rehabilitation program.　1　2　3　4　5　NA

Records and monitors progress of a rehabilitative program.　1　2　3　4　5　NA

Integrates key concepts and skills regarding evaluation and management (eg, therapeutic modalities) of acute and overuse injuries into the rehabilitation program.　1　2　3　4　5　NA

Overall Performance: (choose one)

Outstanding

Very good

Average

Marginal

Unsatisfactory

Describe the student's strengths and/or weaknesses regarding the following areas:

- Accepts and appreciates the roles of allied health professionals.
- Provides education and guidance on preventative techniques specific to the patient population.
- Demonstrates injury evaluation and management skills for injuries/illnesses *specific to the patient population.*
- Utilizes proper treatment, rehabilitation, reconditioning techniques for the injury/illness/condition specific to the patient population.
- Demonstrates an understanding of the organization and administration of sports medicine care delivered in the Rehabilitation clinic and high school settings.
- Demonstrates effective communication skills with patients and allied health professionals.
- Demonstrates an appreciation of diversity and age-group characteristics of the patient population served.
- Understands and identifies clinical outcome assessments through clinician-based (eg, strength, ROM) or patient-based (eg, satisfaction, return to function) measures.
- Additional comments (eg, personal appearance, dependability on completing tasks, quality of work).

Practicum Assignments

High School Rotation Assignments

1st 4-Weeks

ATS completed the Coaches In-Service assignment and discussed this with me.

Yes   No

2nd 4-Weeks

ATS completed the Secondary School Flyer assignment and discussed this with me.

Yes   No

Comments:

REHAB/SPORTS MEDICINE CLINIC ROTATION ASSIGNMENTS

1st 4-Weeks

ATS completed the Medical Abbreviations assignment and discussed this with me.

Yes   No

2nd 4-Weeks

ATS completed the SOAP Notes assignment each week and discussed each with me.

Yes   No

Comments:

Suggested Grade:

A   B   C   D

This report has been discussed with the student: Yes   No

In addition to submitting this evaluation form online, it must be reviewed with the athletic training student. Please print the form, review it with your student, and then both of you sign and date. Have the student submit this completed form to the Program Director. Thanks

Do not type signatures.   Print form first then sign.

Clinical Instructor's Signature: _____

Date: _____

Athletic Training Student's Signature: _____

Date: _____

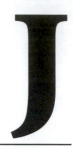

Sample Online Student Clinical Performance Self-Evaluation

Student's Name:

Clinical Assignment:

Current Semester:

DIRECTIONS:

Please evaluate yourself objectively. Check the appropriate response in each category as listed below. Select NA if the item described is not applicable to your clinical experience.

1=Unacceptable   2=Improvement needed   3=Satisfactory   4=Good   5=Outstanding

GENERAL SKILLS AND DUTIES

	1	2	3	4	5	NA
Taping technique	1	2	3	4	5	NA
Treatment technique	1	2	3	4	5	NA
Maintenance of inventory	1	2	3	4	5	NA
Knowledge and implementation of game day procedures	1	2	3	4	5	NA
Sterile technique used when treating wounds	1	2	3	4	5	NA
Does not waste materials	1	2	3	4	5	NA
Is efficient	1	2	3	4	5	NA

Demonstrates initiative	1	2	3	4	5	NA
Involvement in home event coverage	1	2	3	4	5	NA

Comments:

KNOWLEDGE

Recognition of injuries	1	2	3	4	5	NA
Knowledge of injury evaluation techniques	1	2	3	4	5	NA
Obtains correct assessment from injury evaluation	1	2	3	4	5	NA
Knows indications/contraindication	1	2	3	4	5	NA
Knowledge of first aid procedures	1	2	3	4	5	NA
Gives feedback to athlete about progression of their injury	1	2	3	4	5	NA
Willingness to learn	1	2	3	4	5	NA
Inquisitive	1	2	3	4	5	NA

Comments:

ADMINISTRATION TASKS

Knowledge and application of athletic training room procedures	1	2	3	4	5	NA
Knowledge and enforcement of athletic training room policy	1	2	3	4	5	NA
Maintains accurate, current, legible records	1	2	3	4	5	NA
Updates records regularly with progress notes	1	2	3	4	5	NA

Evaluation and rehabilitation reports written
using correct anatomical terminology   1   2   3   4   5   NA

Comments:

INTERPERSONAL SKILLS

ATS demonstrates appropriate communication skills:

Verbal   1   2   3   4   5   NA

Written   1   2   3   4   5   NA

Nonverbal (body language/personal space).   1   2   3   4   5   NA

ATS demonstrates an appropriate level of
empathy with injured patients/athletes.   1   2   3   4   5   NA

ATS is polite in their daily interactions with
supervisors, peers, and patients.   1   2   3   4   5   NA

ATS maintains appropriate boundaries between
personal and clinical experience issues.   1   2   3   4   5   NA

Critical Thinking/Problem Solving   1   2   3   4   5   NA

ATS raises relevant questions with their
clinical supervisor.   1   2   3   4   5   NA

ATS raises questions at an appropriate time.   1   2   3   4   5   NA

ATS is able to recognize problems when they
present.   1   2   3   4   5   NA

Treats patients/athletes without favoritism or
discrimination.   1   2   3   4   5   NA

Comments:

PROFESSIONAL RESPONSIBILITIES

ATS operates within their limitations as they fulfill their clinical experience.	1	2	3	4	5	NA
ATS maintains medical confidentiality at all times.	1	2	3	4	5	NA
ATS is punctual.	1	2	3	4	5	NA
ATS maintains appropriate appearance and dress.	1	2	3	4	5	NA
ATS is willing to do behind the scenes unpleasant duty.	1	2	3	4	5	NA
ATS shows professional honesty and integrity.	1	2	3	4	5	NA
ATS assumes responsibility for learning.	1	2	3	4	5	NA

Comments:

TIME/RESOURCE MANAGEMENT

ATS utilizes clinical supervisor as a resource for questions and problem solving.	1	2	3	4	5	NA
ATS is flexible and can adapt to changes when they present themselves.	1	2	3	4	5	NA
ATS carries out assigned tasks.	1	2	3	4	5	NA
ATS has the capability to multi task while carrying out duties in a clinical setting.	1	2	3	4	5	NA

Comments:

PROFESSIONAL DEVELOPMENT AND INVOLVEMENT

ATS demonstrates a positive attitude toward learning.	1	2	3	4	5	NA

ATS works to put new information into practice.   1   2   3   4   5   NA

ATS fulfills ATEP CEU/In-service obligations.   1   2   3   4   5   NA

Comments:

TECHNICAL STANDARDS

Mental capacity to assimilate, analyze, synthesize,
integrate concepts and problem solve.   1   2   3   4   5   NA

Sufficient postural and neuromuscular control,
sensory function, and coordination to perform
appropriate physical examinations.   1   2   3   4   5   NA

Ability to communicate effectively and sensitively
with patients and colleagues.   1   2   3   4   5   NA

Ability to record the physical examination results
and a treatment plan clearly and accurately.   1   2   3   4   5   NA

Capacity to maintain composure and continue to
function well during periods of high stress.   1   2   3   4   5   NA

Perseverance, diligence and commitment to
complete the athletic training education program. 1   2   3   4   5   NA

Flexibility and the ability to adjust to changing
situations and uncertainty in clinical situations. 1   2   3   4   5   NA

Affective skills and appropriate demeanor and
rapport that relate to professional education
and quality patient care.   1   2   3   4   5   NA

Comments:

LOWER EXTREMITY INJURY ASSESSMENT

Obtains an appropriate medical history of the
patient.   1   2   3   4   5   NA

Performs visual observations of the clinical signs associated with common lower extremity injuries.	1	2	3	4	5	NA
Performs appropriate visual observation of postural, structural and biomechanical abnormalities.	1	2	3	4	5	NA
Palpates the lower extremity bones and soft tissues to determine normal or pathological characteristics.	1	2	3	4	5	NA
Measures the active and passive joint range of motions for the lower extremities.	1	2	3	4	5	NA
Measures resisted manual muscle testing for the lower extremities.	1	2	3	4	5	NA
Applies appropriate lower extremity stress tests for ligamentous or capsular stability.	1	2	3	4	5	NA
Applies appropriate lower extremity special tests.	1	2	3	4	5	NA
Performs an assessment of lower extremity neurological function.	1	2	3	4	5	NA
Documents the results of lower extremity assessments.	1	2	3	4	5	NA

Comments:

Overall strengths:

Overall weaknesses:

Major problem encountered this sport/clinical assignment:

Major goals/objectives to be accomplished during the remainder of sport/clinical assignment:

Additional Comments:

Index

Support your clinical education team...

Is your Clinical Instructor Educator looking for a ready reference to give to Approved Clinical Instructors to help them to deliver a quality educational experience?

The Athletic Trainer's Pocket Guide to Clinical Teaching—now available to buy in quantity for CIEs and ACIs—can help ensure an optimal experience.

Dr. Thomas G. Weidner has created a condensed and well organized book for the *Athletic Training Clinical Education Team* that will provide:

- A general background on effective clinical teaching
- Relevant educational theory
- Specific ideas and strategies for teaching in different clinical settings and situations
- Evaluation and feedback
- Content on how to approach challenges in clinical teaching
- Information for conducting initial and continuing Approved Clinical Instructor (ACI) training

Act now to order multiple copies for your Clinical Education Team

The more you buy—the bigger the discount!

Contact SLACK Incorporated directly for discounts available on the quantity you are interested in purchasing at bookspublishing@slackinc.com

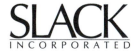